T0235198

CARDIOVASCULAR HAEMODYNAMICS AND DOPPLER WAVEFORMS EXPLAINED

DEDICATION

For Marion, for whom not everything is physics
And Mike Jones, who first enthused me with physics

CARDIOVASCULAR HAEMODYNAMICS AND DOPPLER WAVEFORMS EXPLAINED

Edited by

Crispian Oates

Department of Medical Physics
Regional Physics Department
Newcastle General Hospital
Newcastle upon Tyne

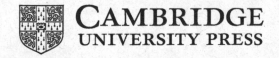

CAMBRIDGE
UNIVERSITY PRESS

CAMBRIDGE UNIVERSITY PRESS
Cambridge, New York, Melbourne, Madrid, Cape Town, Singapore, São Paulo

Cambridge University Press
The Edinburgh Building, Cambridge CB2 8RU, UK

Published in the United States of America by Cambridge University Press, New York

www.cambridge.org
Information on this title: www.cambridge.org/9780521734738

First published 2001
Digitally reprinted by Cambridge University Press 2008

A catalogue record for this publication is available from the British Library

ISBN-13 978-0-521-73473-8 paperback

Every effort has been made in preparing this book to provide accurate and
up-to-date information which is in accord with accepted standards and
practice at the time of publication. Although case histories are drawn
from actual cases, every effort has been made to disguise the identities of
the individuals involved. Nevertheless, the authors, editors and publishers
can make no warranties that the information contained herein is totally
free from error, not least because clinical standards are constantly
changing through research and regulation. The authors, editors and
publishers therefore disclaim all liability for direct or consequential
damages resulting from the use of material contained in this book. Readers
are strongly advised to pay careful attention to information provided by
the manufacturer of any drugs or equipment that they plan to use.

CONTENTS

FOREWORD

This book was written in the hope that it will provide a firm theoretical foundation for those engaged in interpreting Doppler waveforms, whether in cardiac or peripheral vascular work. It was written in the belief that only when one understands the physical principles underlying the patterns of flow seen, and their representation in the form of Doppler waveforms, can a diagnosis of the state of the flow be made with any confidence.

The book divides into three sections. The first two chapters cover the origin and representation of the Doppler waveform. Chapter 1 shows how ultrasound echoes arise from the interaction of ultrasound with blood. Chapter 2 shows how these echoes carry a lot of information about the velocity and motion of the blood that may be displayed as a Doppler spectrum. The importance of the Doppler spectrum is that it is the primary piece of information the operator has to interpret and make measurements from in order to deduce what is going on in the heart and blood vessels of interest. The second section describes the physical process occurring when blood flows around the circulation and the effects that vascular disease has on a normal flow patterns. Chapter 3 covers the basic haemodynamics of flow and chapter 4 discusses the peculiarities of flow that arise as a result of the fact that arterial flow is pulsatile rather than continuous.

The use of ultrasound to investigate disease in the circulation differs from that of other organs because the "organ of interest", the cardiovascular system, is extended throughout the body and is dynamic system. As an example, when the kidney is examined, it is seen within the ultrasound image together with any abnormalities that may be present. Virtually all the relevant information from kidney is seen in the image before the operator. In contrast, the state of blood flow to the lower limb not only depends on the section of vessel that is seen, but also depends on the function of the heart, the arteries proximal to the point of observation and the condition of the distil circulation. These all affect the waveforms that are seen. Because of the linear nature of the circulation a segmental approach to scanning blood vessels is often adopted. Each vessel segment is examined in turn. If a normal waveform is seen entering a segment and a normal waveform is seen leaving a segment, it may usually be concluded that there is no significant disease within the segment. This approach is particularly useful where it is not possible to view a particular section of vessel directly.

Having obtained a Doppler waveform, the process of interpretation is essentially one of pattern recognition and is founded on the basis that each normal range of waveforms that will change in the presence of disease. In order to fully understand these changes, it is important to know how the whole cardiovascular systems works as well as understanding the local effects of cardiovascular disease. Background knowledge of the whole system also shows the inter-relationship between the work of the heart and the circulation it supplies, and enables one to understand how physical changes in the system produce clinical changes and symptoms that cause patients to be referred for cardiovascular investigation. The operator will then have insight into the flow patterns that might be expected in normal and pathological conditions. This can be very useful when considering differential diagnosis and when something new or unexpected is seen. The third section is therefore included to give an overview of the haemodynamic function of the heart circulation. Chapter 5 considers the function of the heart and what happens when it fails. Chapter 6 looks at the circulation and its control in maintaining an adequate oxygen supply to all tissues under the changing metabolic demands. The effects of aging and disease are described.

Throughout the book specific clinical application of the theory being discussed is highlighted in boxes separated from the main text. A number of technical notes are also put in this form. The practice of vascular ultrasound and echocardiography has developed immensely in the last 20 years, since the early attempts to interpret what was seen and heard. They are now firmly established as clinical investigations that have an important role to play in patient management. If this book enables those practising in the profession to improve their understanding technique and confidence in diagnosis, so enabling the cardiovascular use of ultrasound to develop and move on to the benefit of patients, then it will have achieved its purpose.

ACKNOWLEDGEMENTS

The writing of this book has greatly benefited from the help, feedback and encouragement of many friends and colleagues. It all began with the students in my vascular course under whose auspices the inspiration for the book was born. Mark Haines, John Hay and Susanna Oates very kindly acted as the models for many of the normal waveforms. Dr Zaw Htet, Dr Stewart Hunter, Alison Heads and her colleagues gave much valuable advice on the cardiac aspects of the book and professor Robert Wilkinson and Dr Iain Chambers kindly contributed to the description of control of total blood volume and cerebral perfusion respectively. Dr Simon Elliott advised and encouraged through many discussions and kindly contributed the images for figure 6.22. John Allen helped with the information on the microcirculation and gave the data for figure 6.20. Many helpful comments have been made by my colleagues in the vascular laboratory and the patients passing through have provided many of the images as we sought to investigate and help their condition. As a constant inspiration and help in all matters ultrasonic I must thank Dr Tony Whittingham and for everything else I have to thank my very tolerant wife, Marion.

These all have helped in the making of the book, however I am responsible for the content and any mistakes are undoubtedly mine.

Crispian Oates

1

BLOOD – THE ULTRASOUND TARGET OF INTEREST

Echogenicity of blood

Composition of blood

Origin of echoes from blood

BLOOD – THE ULTRASOUND TARGET OF INTEREST

Outline

The chapter shows where echoes arising from blood originate and describes how they vary depending on the physical conditions in the blood target.

For Doppler ultrasound investigations, blood is the ultrasound target of interest. The echoes received from blood contain all the information for the scanner to display velocity waveforms so that the operator can assess the haemodynamic status of the vessels. We therefore begin by looking at the interaction of ultrasound with blood as an echogenic target.

The strength of the signal received by the ultrasound transducer will depend on the backscattering of ultrasound by blood and attenuation of the ultrasound by intervening tissue. Compared with adjacent tissues such as muscle, the echogenicity of blood is very low. For example, there is a difference of 43 dB in the echo strength between muscle and blood. The lumen of an artery or heart chamber therefore appears dark on a B-mode image. Some ultrasound scanners with a large dynamic range do show a faint speckle pattern within the vessel lumen. In addition to the greater echogenicity of surrounding tissue, the vessel wall itself forms a strong specular reflector when viewed at 90° to the direction of the propagation of ultrasound. The wall then appears as a bright structure that may produce reverberations on the B-mode image which extend into the lumen. Specular reflection by the vessel wall also reduces the intensity I_t of the ultrasound transmitted into the lumen, thus reducing the returning signal strength still further. This problem is made worse when the vessel walls have become calcified with disease and when the vessel is viewed obliquely to give a good Doppler angle θ_D (Figure 1.1).

The relative backscatter of blood, skeletal muscle and liver at 5 MHz is shown in Table 1.1.

Table 1.1 – Relative backscatter of blood, skeletal muscle and liver at 5 MHz

Tissue	Relative backscatter (cm⁻¹ Sr⁻¹)
Blood	76.9×10^{-6}
Skeletal muscle	10.4×10^{-3}
Liver	2.9×10^{-3}

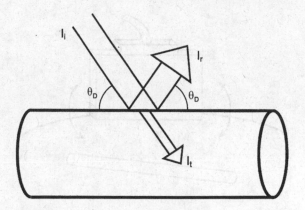

Figure 1.1 – A large reflection of an ultrasound beam at a vessel wall (θ_D) with a reduced intensity penetrating the vessel lumen (I_t). I_i, incident intensity; I_r, intensity reflected at the vessel wall.

Clinical note
Obtaining a good Doppler signal when echo strength is poor

Optimising the scanner settings when the Doppler signal strength is poor requires ensuring that the maximum transmitted pulse enters the vessel and that the sensitivity in detection is maximised. A low Doppler transmitted frequency should be used, possibly by using a low-frequency probe. Sensitivity will be greatest when the ultrasound beam is directed in a forward direction at 90° to the transducer face. Penetration of ultrasound into the vessel lumen is better when the vessel axis is at 90° to the direction of the ultrasound beam (Figure 1.1). For this reason, in situations where the signal strength is poor, a high Doppler angle may have to be used even though it leads to a poor estimation of true velocity. Colour sensitivity is improved by using a low-velocity scale, even if this produces aliasing. Both colour and Doppler gain should be increased until noise appears and then slightly backed-off.

The following guidelines may help in obtaining a useful signal:

- Set the angle of the colour Doppler box to be nearly perpendicular to the vessel axis and try using a low-velocity scale or power Doppler to improve the colour filling of the lumen. The sensitivity of the transducer will be greatest when the colour box or pulsed-Doppler beam

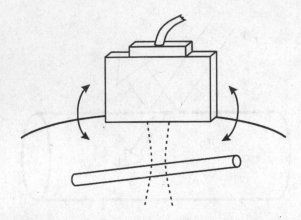

Figure 1.2 – 'Heel and toe' movement of an ultrasound transducer on the skin surface to obtain an acceptable Doppler angle.

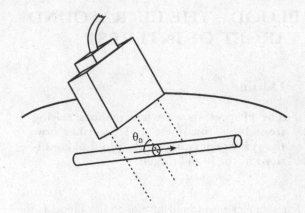

Figure 1.3 – An ultrasound transducer positioned to obtain a transverse view of a vessel with a Doppler angle θ_D.

is at 90° to the transducer face. A Doppler angle may then be produced by 'heel and toe' movements of the probe on the skin surface (Figure 1.2).

- When there is extensive calcification, the colour signal may be patchy along the line of the vessel. Place the Doppler sample volume for pulsed–Doppler over an area of good colour signal. The Doppler waveforms should then also be of good quality.

- In the absence of any colour filling of the vessel lumen, place the pulsed–Doppler sample volume over the position of the vessel on the B-mode image and attempt to obtain a Doppler signal.

- When visualisation on B-mode and colour Doppler is poor, vessels may appear more clearly on the B-mode image when viewed in transverse section with the colour box set to 90° to the transducer surface (Figure 1.3). As

long as the transducer is tilted along the line of the vessel, a Doppler signal may still be obtained. The Doppler angle, θ_D, will be unknown and so no velocity measurements can be made, but vessel patency and waveform shape may be assessed.

Echogenicity of blood.

Blood is an inhomogeneous liquid. It consists of a suspension of cells and other particles in plasma, which is a clear straw-coloured fluid. These components between them form a fine microscopic structure that can scatter ultrasound to produce the echoes detected. The particulate components of blood are erythrocytes or red blood cells (RBC), leukocytes or white blood cells (WBC) and platelets. In normal blood they are present in the concentrations shown in Table 1.2.

RBC have the shape of a disc with concave surfaces measuring 7.5 μm wide by 2.2 μm thick (Figure 1.4).

Table 1.2 – Properties of normal blood and its constituents

	Dimensions (μm)	Concentration (particles mm⁻³)	Percentage of total blood volume	Density, ρ (kg m⁻³)	Compressibility, β (m² N⁻¹)	Acoustic impedance, Z_0 (kg m⁻² s⁻¹)
Whole blood	–	–	100	1060	–	–
Plasma	–	–	54	1027	4.09×10^{-10}	1.58×10^6
RBC	7.5×2.2	5×10^6	45	1093	3.41×10^{-10}	1.79×10^6
WBC	9–25	8×10^3	~0.8	–	–	–
Platelets	2–3	3.5×10^5	~0.2	–	–	–

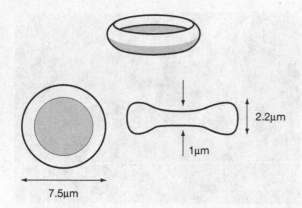

Figure 1.4 – Shape and dimensions of a red blood cell.

The large number and size of RBC means that they are almost entirely responsible for the scattering of ultrasound within blood. The fact that ultrasound is scattered by RBC at all is due to the difference in density and compressibility between them and plasma, that is, there is a difference in acoustic impedance. The percentage volume of whole blood occupied by RBC is known as the **haematocrit**. In normal blood the haematocrit is 45% for men and 42% for women, but these values may vary significantly with disease, from 9% in severe anaemia to > 70% in polycythaemia. The way RBC interact with each other affects the strength of the ultrasound signal received by the transducer. These interactions depend upon the haematocrit, the presence of fibrinogen, a large protein molecule in plasma, and for turbulent flow, the density difference between RBC and plasma.

The wavelength of ultrasound over the range of frequencies used in diagnostic ultrasound, 2–10 MHz, is 0.79–0.16 mm. As the size of the scatterer is very much less than these wavelengths, **Rayleigh scattering** occurs. Energy from the ultrasound pulse will be scattered in all directions. The transducer only receives the portion of scattered energy that is scattered back towards it. For Rayleigh scattering, the factors affecting the **backscattered power** P_{BS} reaching the transducer are, the number of scatterers n in the sample volume V which depends on the pulse shape, the intensity I_i of the incident ultrasound frequency f, the radius of scatterer a, the distance of the target from the transducer r, and a factor $s(k\rho)$ involving the compressibility k and density ρ of plasma and RBC:

$$P_{BS} \propto \frac{n V I_i a^6 f^4 s\,(k\rho)}{r^2}$$

The Scattering Equation

Note:

- There is a strong dependence on the ultrasound frequency (f^4). A higher frequency transducer will give a stronger Doppler signal for a given incident intensity. In practice this will be offset by the increased attenuation of a higher frequency ultrasound beam by the intervening tissue.

- The signal strength will depend on the size and number of scatterers.

- There is a very strong dependence on scatterer size (a^6).

Composition of blood

Figure 1.5 shows how the backscattered power from blood varies with haematocrit. At low haematocrits of < 10% the RBC act as independent scatterers. Their concentration in plasma is then so low that they do not stay in contact with each other for very long when they collide. The scattering equation shows that as the number of RBC increases from zero, the Doppler signal should linearly increase in strength. The scatterer size will be the RBC mean diameter, 2.75 μm.

As the haematocrit increases above ~10%, there are enough RBC present to form groups of cells that act as larger scatterers. This is in addition to the many single-cell scatterers present. The larger scatterers will give a larger signal. Their number increases as the haematocrit increases and the increase in Doppler signal strength is then no longer linear.

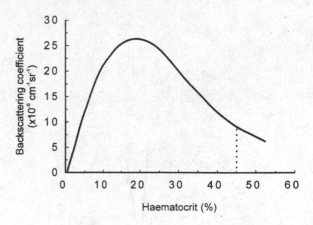

Figure 1.5 – Change in the backscattered ultrasound signal against haematocrit. Results are obtained from human red blood cells with uniform flow.[1]

At physiological haematocrits, there are so many RBC present that they can no longer be considered individually. At a haematocrit of 45% the average gap between each RBC is only 10% of each RBC's diameter. The RBC concentration is then so high that the scatterers may be thought of as plasma 'holes' in a continuum of RBC (Figure 1.6). As the haematocrit increases to its upper limit of ~70%, the Doppler signal decreases as the number and size of plasma holes decreases.

Origin of echoes from blood

There are three situations where the echogenicity of blood is increased.

Stationary blood

At very low velocities when the velocity gradient, or sheer rate, across the vessel is low, the 'discs' of RBC adhere to one another to form multicellular clumps called **rouleaux** (Figure 1.7).

These form scattering centres that are much larger than the normal variations in cell–plasma densities and may be a significant proportion of a wavelength in size. The rouleaux therefore give a much larger backscattered echo and produce a distinct fine speckle pattern on a B-mode image. This speckle pattern becomes apparent within a few seconds of the blood coming to rest as occurs, for example, in some large veins. It is also sometimes seen in the heart when wall movement is reduced due to infarction when it appears as a 'wisp of smoke' during

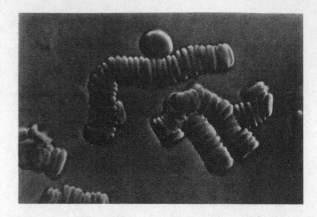

Figure 1.7 – Profile view of red blood cells stacking up to form rouleaux.[2]

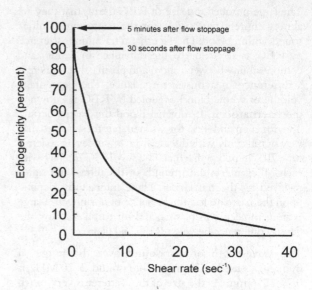

Figure 1.8 – Echogenicity of human blood against shear rate relative to echogenicity 5 min after flow stoppage.[3]

part of the cardiac cycle. As soon as the blood starts to move again the rouleaux break-up and the speckle pattern vanishes. Figure 1.8 shows how the echogenicity of blood increases as the shear rate decreases.

Turbulent flow

In the complex motion of turbulent flow, the plasma and RBC are pulled apart from one another to produce larger-scale density variations in the matrix of RBC in plasma. This is due to the accelerations and

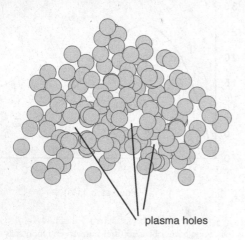

Figure 1.6 – 'Plasma holes' in a matrix of red blood cells.

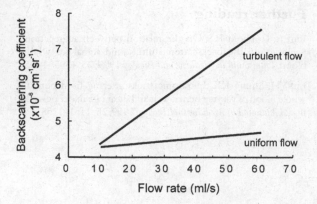

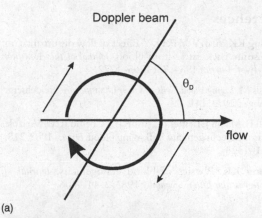

(a)

Figure 1.9 – Increase in echogenicity with turbulent blood flow. Measurements were made with bovine red blood cell suspension at 40% haematocrit.[1]

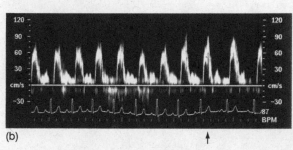

(b)

changes of direction seen in turbulence producing inertial forces that act on the density difference between RBC and plasma. These larger-scale variations in density give rise to a larger backscattered echo as the effective scatterer size is increased (Figure 1.9).

A special case of this phenomenon is seen when a discrete vortex forms within the flow (Figure 1.10a). The vortex travels down the vessel as a large self-contained structure that gives a strong echo. It also produces higher Doppler frequencies than the surrounding blood as it has components at a Doppler angle, θ_D, of zero. Such vortices show themselves on the Doppler waveform as spike turbulence (Figure 1.10b). They are also seen in turbulent flow in the heart chambers as distinct bright speckles appearing on the B-mode image.

Figure 1.10 – (a) How an increased Doppler signal arises from a vortex moving along in the blood-flow. Higher Doppler frequencies are detected from components of flow at a Doppler angle, θ_D, of zero; (b) example of spike turbulence on an aortic waveform.

Thrombus

When a thrombus forms within a vessel lumen or heart chamber, the lumen becomes echogenic. In the acute phase a venous thrombus is strongly echogenic. At 24 h it becomes less echogenic again, probably due to cross-linking of fibrin and the development of zones of haemolysis. Within a few days a heterogeneous appearance is seen as the thrombus retracts and echogenicity continues to increase. The exact course of the changes in echogenicity varies considerably and the dating of thrombosis by these appearances is not very reliable. These changes are indicated in Figure 1.11.

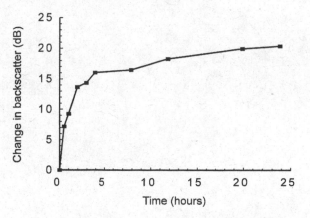

Figure 1.11 – Change in ultrasound backscatter from a unit volume of blood during coagulation. Measurements were made with human blood at 44% haematocrit.[4]

References

1. Shung KK, Yuan YW, Fei DY. Effect of flow disturbance on ultrasonic backscatter from blood. *Journal of the Acoustical Society of America* 1984; **75**: 1265–1272.

2. Bessis M. *Living Blood Cells and their Ultrastructure.* Heidelberg: Springer, 1973: 141.

3. Sigel B, Machi J, Beitler JC, Justin JR, Coelho JCU. Variable ultrasound echogenicity in flowing blood. *Science* 1982; **218**: 1321–1323.

4. Shung KK. Physics of blood echogenicity. *Journal of Cardiovascular Ultrasonography* 1983; **2**: 401–406.

Further reading

Lim B, Cobbold RS. On the relation between aggregation, packing and the backscattered ultrasound signal for whole blood. *Ultrasound in Medicine and Biology* 1999; **25**: 1395–1405.

Lin YH, Shung KK. Ultrasonic backscattering from porcine whole blood of varying hematocrit and shear rate under pulsatile flow. *Ultrasound in Medicine and Biology* 1999; **25**: 1151–1158.

2

WHAT THE DOPPLER SPECTRAL WAVEFORM SHOWS

Doppler equation

Doppler power spectrum

Doppler waveforms

Doppler waveform measurements

Doppler waveform artefacts

Colour-flow imaging

Power Doppler

WHAT THE DOPPLER SPECTRAL WAVEFORM SHOWS

Outline

The chapter describes the origin of the Doppler equation and shows how the Doppler spectrum is formed. Measurements from the Doppler waveform are discussed and artefacts that may occur illustrated. The use of colour-flow imaging is discussed.

For a stationary ultrasound target, the frequency of echoes returning to the ultrasound transducer will equal the transmitted frequency f_T. This is not the case for a moving target such as blood. For a target moving towards the transducer, the frequency of returning echoes f_R will be higher than f_T, and for a target moving away f_R will be lower than f_T. This change in received frequency for echoes from moving blood is an occurrence of the phenomenon called the **Doppler effect**. It may be explained by considering the process of transmission of ultrasound and backscattering by the moving target in two parts.

The Doppler Equation

First of all we look at what an observer standing on a target red blood cell (RBC) sees as the RBC moves towards the transducer (Figure 2.1). In this situation, the transmitter is stationary and the RBC is a moving receiver. The speed of sound in blood is $c = 1570$ ms^{-1} and may be considered constant. The wavelength λ and frequency of sound f are related by:

$$c = f\lambda.$$

Let f_T be the frequency transmitted by the transducer. Because the RBC is moving towards the oncoming wavefronts, it encounters successive wave crests at an increased frequency. This can be thought of as due to an apparent change in the speed of sound caused by the velocity v of the RBC so that the frequently f_T' seen by the RBC is given by:

$$f_T' = \frac{(c+v)}{\lambda_T} = f_T \frac{(c+v)}{c} = f_T\left(1+\frac{v}{c}\right)$$

So the increase in detected frequency at the RBC is $\frac{v}{c}$

In the second part the RBC re-transmits the sound waves as a backscattered echo towards the transducer so there is now a moving transmitter and a stationary receiver (Figure 2.2).

Between transmitting each wavefront at f_T', the RBC runs onto the previously transmitted wavefront to shorten the wavelength λ_R travelling back to the transducer. As above, this wavelength change is related to an apparent change in the speed of sound, so:

$$\lambda_R = \frac{(c-v)}{f_T'} = \frac{c}{f_R} \quad \text{or} \quad f_R = f_T' \frac{1}{\left(1-\frac{v}{c}\right)}$$

where f_R is the frequency received by the transducer. Using the fact that the blood velocities encountered in the body, v is very much less than c, this can be rearranged as follows:

$$f_R = f_T' \frac{\left(1+\frac{v}{c}\right)}{\left(1+\frac{v}{c}\right)} \cdot \frac{1}{\left(1-\frac{v}{c}\right)} = f_T' \frac{\left(1+\frac{v}{c}\right)}{\left(1+\frac{v^2}{c^2}\right)} \approx f_T'\left(1+\frac{v}{c}\right)$$

as $\frac{v^2}{c^2}$ is negligibly small and can be ignored. The increase in detected frequency at the transducer is therefore seen to be $\frac{v}{c}$ again. Putting the outward and

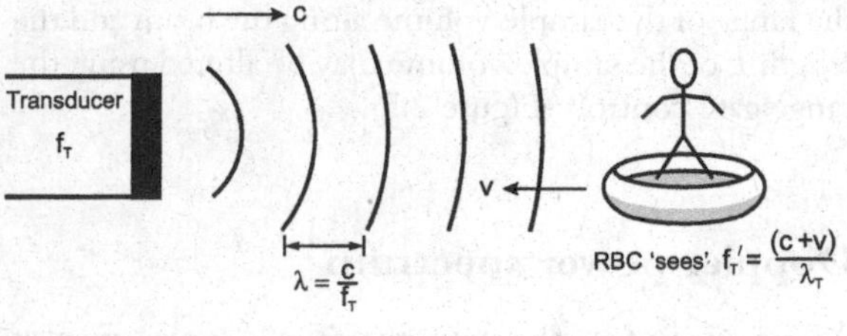

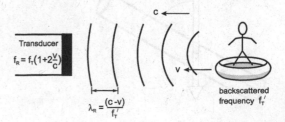

Figure 2.1 – Diagram showing derivation of Doppler equation.

Figure 2.2 – Second diagram for deriving Doppler equation.

return journeys together by substituting for $f_T{}'$, and again ignoring $\frac{v^2}{c^2}$, we have:

$$f_R = f_T\left(1+\frac{v}{c}\right)\left(1+\frac{v}{c}\right) = f_T\left(1+2\frac{v}{c}+\frac{v^2}{c^2}\right) \approx f_T\left(1+2\frac{v}{c}\right)$$

The Doppler shift or **Doppler frequency** is the difference between the transmitted and received frequencies so:

$$f_R - f_T = f_D = f_T 2\frac{v}{c}$$

and the factor 2 is seen to be due to there being a Doppler shift on the outward journey with a second shift on the return journey. This equation has been arrived at by considering flow directly towards the transducer. A similar argument for a target moving directly away from the transducer gives a reduction in received frequency:

$$f_R - f_T\left(1-2\frac{v}{c}\right)$$

Where flow is in some other direction at an angle θ_D towards the transducer, the proportion of motion towards the transducer is given by $\cos(\theta_D)$ (Figure 2.3). θ_D is called the **Doppler angle**. The general relationship between the Doppler frequency and target velocity is therefore:

$$f_D = 2\frac{v}{c}f_T\cos(\theta_D)$$

The Doppler Equation

The Doppler frequency will be maximum for $\theta_D = 0°$ ($\cos\theta = 1$) when blood flow direction is exactly in line with the ultrasound beam and will be zero for $\theta_D = 90°$ ($\cos\theta = 0$).

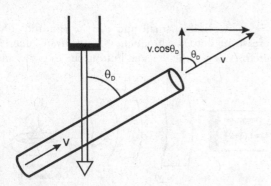

Figure 2.3 – Derivation of the $v\cos(\theta_D)$ component of velocity towards the transducer.

There are only a few places in the body where an angle of zero degrees between the flow and the ultrasound beam may be achieved. On duplex scanners that combine both B-mode imaging and pulsed-Doppler, the Doppler angle may be determined from the B-mode image by aligning the angle cursor on the image parallel to the direction of blood flow (Figure 2.9). The Doppler angle is then known and the Doppler equation may be solved to give blood velocities.

Clinical note
Doppler angle

In general the smallest Doppler angle consistent with maintaining adequate signal strength should be used. This will give the greatest Doppler frequency f_D and hence sensitivity to low velocity flows. On duplex scanners this may be achieved by steering the Doppler beam and tilting the transducer from end to end within the scan plane, a procedure known as 'heel and toeing' the probe (Figure 1.2). When making velocity measurements from Doppler waveforms, the Doppler angle should be $\leq 60°$. At higher angles the error in calculating the flow velocity due to small errors in angle measurements becomes unacceptably high. Figure 2.4 shows the error in $\cos\theta$ for a 2° error in measuring the Doppler angle.

For a single target moving with velocity v, the Doppler equation gives the relationship between the Doppler frequency and that velocity. In any blood vessel there will be many such targets having many different velocities and these will give a range or **spectrum of Doppler frequencies**. The Doppler frequencies actually detected will arise from targets lying within the sensitive **sample volume** of the ultrasound beam. For continuous-wave Doppler probes, the sample volume is fixed by the geometrical arrangement of the transducer elements. For pulsed-Doppler probes, both the range of the sample volume along the beam and the length L of the sample volume may be altered using the range gate controls (Figure 2.5).

Doppler power spectrum

At any one instant, the strength of the Doppler signal at each Doppler frequency may be plotted as shown for

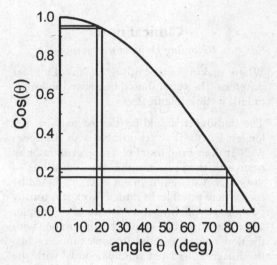

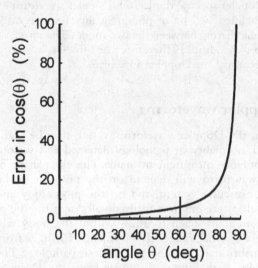

Figure 2.4 – Effect on cos (θ) of a 2° error in measuring the Doppler angle (θ). Measurements made using θ ≤ 60° will have an acceptably small error if θ is carefully measured.

two examples in Figure 2.6. This is known as an **instantaneous Doppler power spectrum**. The amount of blood moving at each velocity within the sample volume determines the value of the curve at each corresponding Doppler frequency.

The plots shown therefore give a picture of the instantaneous distribution of velocities amongst all the targets within the sample volume. Figure 2.6(a) shows that nearly all the blood is moving in a narrow range of high velocities with very little moving at low velocities. At some time later the distribution of velocities may have

changed to be like that shown in Figure 2.6(b). Now, instead of most of the blood moving at a high velocity, we see that the blood flow is evenly distributed across a wide range of velocities. The area under each curve is the same and is proportional to the total backscattered

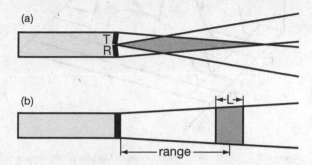

Figure 2.5 – Sample volume (deeply shaded area) for (a) a continuous-wave Doppler transducer with separate transmit and receive elements and (b) a pulsed-wave Doppler transducer in which the received signal is range-gated so as to admit echoes over a length L.

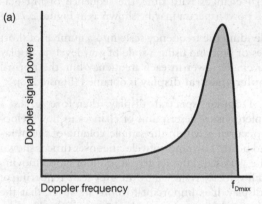

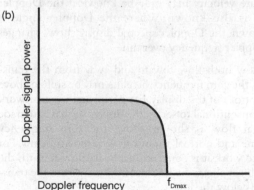

Figure 2.6 – Two instantaneous Doppler power spectra arising from different velocity distributions within the same vessel at different times. The area under each curve is the same.

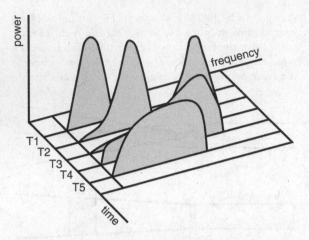

Figure 2.7 – Five consecutive instantaneous Doppler power spectra arranged to show the change in velocity distribution with time.

power which depends on the total number of targets within the sample volume. To observe how the flow pattern changes with time, the sequence of instantaneous power spectra may be shown as in Figure 2.7.

By dividing the frequency scale into a number of short ranges or bins and using a scale of grey levels to display the average power in each frequency bin, the normal **Doppler spectral display** is obtained (Figure 2.8).

The Doppler spectral display therefore gives a complete visual description of changes in flow velocities occurring within the sample volume of the ultrasound beam. The range of velocities over time is shown on the y-axis and the relative amount of blood moving at each velocity is shown by the grey scale rendering of the display. It is important to note, however, that the absolute velocity may only be known if the Doppler angle is also known. Where the Doppler angle is unknown, the Doppler spectral display shows changes in Doppler frequency over time.

To show both flow toward and away from the transducer, the zero frequency baseline may be shifted above the bottom of the display. For peripheral vascular work it is conventional to set up the display so that antegrade arterial flow is shown above the zero frequency baseline and normal venous flow is shown below. For cardiac work it is conventional to set flow towards the transducer above the line and flow away from the transducer below the line.

For convenience the Doppler spectral display is usually referred to as simply the **Doppler spectrum**. The flow patterns displayed are called **Doppler waveforms**.

Doppler waveforms

From the Doppler waveforms, vessels may be identified, normality or pathology detected and various quantitative measurements made. The exact shape of the waveform will depend on the position in the cardiovascular system, and on the physiology and pathology present proximally, distally or at the site of measurement. Each location within the body will have a normal range of waveforms. Changes from normality may be used to diagnose pathology. The process of making a diagnosis from the Doppler waveform is mainly one of pattern recognition together with an understanding of what causes the particular waveform shape to occur. Quantitative measurements may be made to confirm and categorise the waveform types seen. Consider first the process of pattern recognition. The human visual cortex is very adept at recognising features of interest within a complex image. An experienced operator can often make a competent diagnosis by simple visual inspection of the waveform. Learning to recognise which are the informative features and recognising subtle differences between waveforms may take a considerable time to achieve. In the end, there is no substitute for seeing lots of cases. They should be reviewed together with a more experienced operator or compared with some other

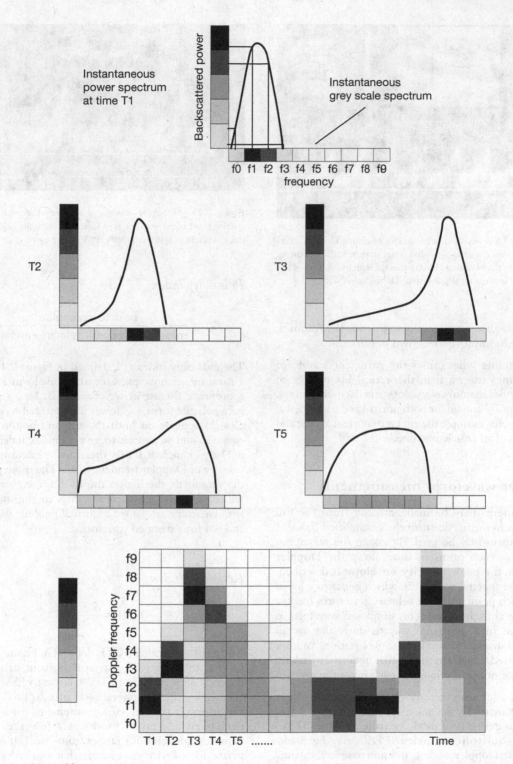

Figure 2.8 – Rendering of five consecutive Doppler power spectra using a grey scale to indicate power and then their arrangement to form the familiar Doppler spectral display.

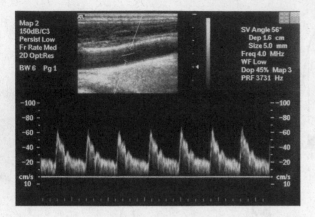

Figure 2.9 – Ideal way to view a vessel for obtaining Doppler wave-forms. The vessel is imaged with a long, straight section showing bright walls as the ultrasound beam passes through its centre line. The angle cursor is correctly aligned parallel to the vessel walls.

modality such as angiography to provide the feedback necessary to improve one's own performance.

Understanding what causes the particular waveform shape comes from a firm theoretical knowledge of cardiovascular anatomy, physiology and haemodynamics. These must be known for both normal and pathological conditions, for example the effects of normal ageing and the effects of atherosclerotic disease.

Doppler waveform measurements

Measurements may be made directly from the full spectral waveform. Alternatively a simplified form of the waveform may be used. By taking the maximum velocity at each point in time along the Doppler waveform, the **peak velocity envelope** is described. Unlike the spectral waveform, which contains a lot of data at each point, the peak velocity waveform has just one value at each instant. This simplified waveform is often used in a shorthand way to show the overall waveform shape obtained from some location. Another single-valued waveform used is that obtained by taking the average or mean velocity at each instant in time.

The peak and mean velocity waveforms can be calculated automatically on most scanners (Figure 2.10). Spot measurements of **peak systolic velocity** (PSV) and **end-diastolic velocity** (EDV) may be made. Where the Doppler angle is unknown, several quantitative indices have been devised that enable cos (θ_D) in the Doppler equation to be eliminated.

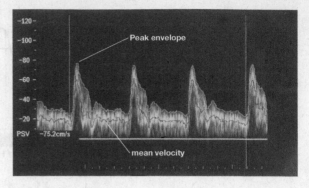

Figure 2.10 – Doppler waveform showing the peak velocity envelope and mean velocity waveform automatically calculated by the scanner. Peak systolic velocity (PSV) is also given.

Pulsatility index

$$PI = \frac{\text{peak to peak value}}{\text{mean value of peak velocity envelope}}$$

The pulsatility index (PI; defined in Figure 2.11) gives a measure of how pulsatile the waveform is and is appropriate for use in waveforms that have a particularly pulsatile form, e.g. lower limb arterial waveforms. Cos (θ) appears on both the top and bottom of the equation and so cancels to give an index independent of Doppler angle θ. It may therefore be calculated using velocity or Doppler frequency data. The more pulsatile the waveform, the higher the PI. Damped waveforms will have a low PI. Typical values in the superficial femoral artery are 10 for a normal pulsatile waveform and < 4 for a damped waveform.

Resistance index

$$RI = \frac{A - B}{A}$$

The resistance index (RI) is defined in Figure 2.12. As for PI, the cos (θ)'s top and bottom cancel. RI depends on a changing EDV relative to PSV. EDV is affected by the peripheral resistance to flow seen by the artery at the site of measurement. An increased peripheral resistance produces a lower EDV, and hence a higher RI. RI ranges from 0 to 1. It is appropriate for use in waveforms that normally have a continuous forward flow throughout diastole, for example carotid arteries.

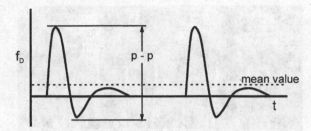

Figure 2.11 – Definition of the pulsatility index (PI).

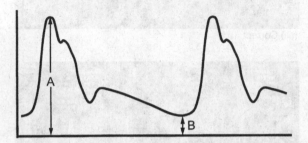

Figure 2.12 – Peak systolic velocity (A) and end–diastolic velocity (B) used to calculate the resistance index (RI).

A closely related index to RI is the **A/B ratio** (Figure 2.12):

$$A/B \text{ ratio} = \frac{A}{B}$$

The ratio has been used to measure changes in peripheral resistance in organs such as the placenta and transplanted liver.

Systolic rise time (SRT) may be measured in milliseconds directly from the Doppler waveform. It provides a quantitative measurement of waveform damping that occurs when flow in an artery is maximal, usually as a result of severe proximal disease (Figure 2.13).

Other indices and mathematical analyses of the Doppler waveforms have been used with varying degrees of success or proven usefulness. Some of those used are site specific and will be described as those clinical areas are discussed (see Further reading). Most modern scanners have calculation packages that automatically produce the standard measurements and indices from the waveforms.

Clinical note
Optimising the display of a Doppler spectrum

To optimise the display of arterial Doppler waveforms when making measurements, the velocity scale and baseline position should be adjusted so that the whole waveform is seen and the peak systolic velocity is displayed at the maximum size possible (Figure 2.14a).

For measurements of systolic rise time, the display sweep speed should be set to its maximum rate to give the best temporal resolution (Figure 2.14b). The gain applied to the Doppler signal should ideally be set to clearly show the peak velocity outline of the waveform compatible with not over-amplifying background noise. Where the signal is very noisy the operator must manually position the callipers to make measurements and must not rely on the automatic calculation of parameters by the scanner to find PSV, EDV, etc. correctly. Where an automatic calculation package is used, the values obtained should be visually checked to ensure they are correct.

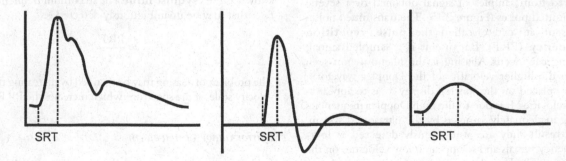

Figure 2.13 – Cursor positions used for calculating systolic rise time (SRT) for three waveforms.

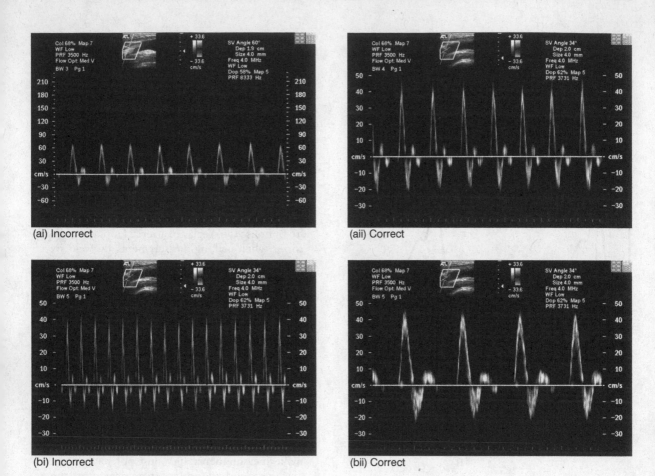

Figure 2.14 – Correct way (aii, bii) to set up the velocity scale to make full use of the scanner velocity sensitivity and (ai, bi) to set up the sweep speed to make time measurements such as systolic rise time with the best time resolution.

Doppler waveform artefacts

Aliasing

When using pulsed-Doppler, the Doppler frequency is derived from samples of signal obtained over several transmitted pulses (Figure 2.15). The transmitted pulses are sent at a rate called the **pulse repetition frequency** (PRF). Because it is a sampled signal, aliasing can occur. Aliasing is the phenomenon seen when the higher velocities of the Doppler waveform are misplaced on the spectral display so as to appear as low velocities. It is due to the high Doppler frequencies being inadequately sampled by the ultrasound system. As a result they are ambiguously detected as low-frequency signals and so appear as low velocities on the spectrum. The Doppler waveform then appears to 'wrap around' the spectrum (Figure 2.16). To unambiguously

determine a Doppler frequency, there must be at least two samples within one cycle of the Doppler signal (Figure 2.15). That is, at least two samples are required to know that the amplitude has oscillated above and below zero within the time interval of one period. This is known as the **Nyquist limit**. The maximum frequency $f_{D\,max}$ that may be unambiguously detected is:

$$f_{Dmax} = \frac{PRF}{2}$$

The problem of aliasing may be rectified by increasing the velocity scale of the spectrum which increases the PRF.

Mirror image of waveform

In the mirror-image artefact shown in Figure 2.17 an exact copy of the true waveform appears as a reflection

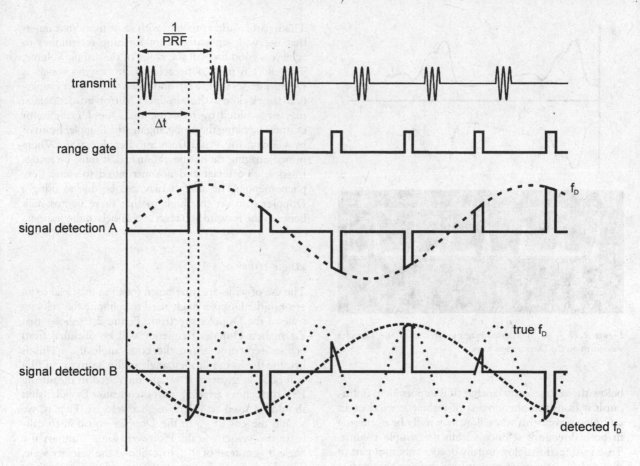

Figure 2.15 – For pulsed-Doppler it is shown (A) how the Doppler frequency is derived from a sampled signal and (B) how it can be ambiguously detected causing aliasing if the sample rate is too low.

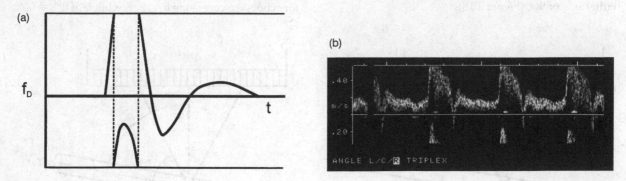

Figure 2.16 – (a, b) Appearance of aliasing on the Doppler spectrum showing that high Doppler frequencies are detected and displayed as low frequencies.

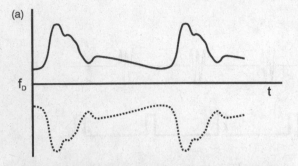

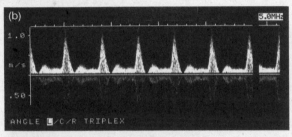

Figure 2.17 – (a, b) Mirror-imaging artefact of the Doppler waveform on the Doppler spectrum.

below the zero velocity baseline. It is important to distinguish it from the phenomena of turbulence and other complex waveforms when flow may really be occurring in both directions at once within the sample volume. True bi-directional flow usually occurs only over part of the cardiac cycle, whereas in mirror imaging the artefact is seen throughout the cardiac cycle. It is usually caused when the Doppler ultrasound beam and sample volume are positioned so that Doppler angles to the flow exist either side of 90° (Figure 2.18).

This is particularly a problem with some modern scanners that use wide-aperture beam-forming techniques to achieve a good focus at the range of the sample volume. The effect is most noticeable when viewing vessels at Doppler angles near to 90° and when viewing very superficial vessels close to the transducer. Mirror-image artefacts may be avoided by reducing the Doppler angle, for example by tilting the probe, angling the Doppler beam or by viewing the vessel from another direction. Where mirror imaging cannot be eliminated, it must be recognised as an artefact and not attributed to some flow phenomenon. The artefact may also be due to using a Doppler gain set too high so that there is cross-talk between the forward and reverse channels in the scanner.

Angle error

The use of wide-aperture beam forming may lead to an error in the Doppler angle used to calibrate the velocity scale of the Doppler spectrum. Figure 2.19 shows that the highest Doppler frequency will be obtained from echoes returning along the edge angle θ_{edge}. This is because θ_{edge} is the smallest angle in the beam so cos (θ_D) will be at its greatest. If we are interested in measuring PSV, the echoes arriving with the greatest Doppler shift should be used to calculate that velocity. That is, we should use cos (θ_{edge}) in the Doppler equation to calibrate the velocity scale. However, some scanners use angle θ_{mid} instead of θ_{edge} to calibrate the velocity scale. This leads to an over estimation of peak velocities because echoes from θ_{edge} will have a higher Doppler frequency than those from θ_{mid} and will therefore be displayed at a higher velocity on the scale that reads true for echoes arriving along θ_{mid}. For example, if $\theta_{mid} = 60°$,

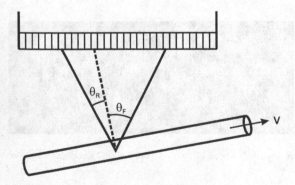

Figure 2.18 – How a mirror-imaging artefact arises from a wide ultrasound beam having angular components on both sides of a line perpendicular to the direction of target movement.

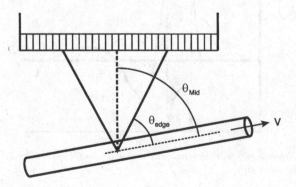

Figure 2.19 – Two Doppler angles that may be used by a scanner to calculate the velocity scale. Use of the wrong angle can lead to errors in velocity measurements.

θ_{edge} = 50°, true blood velocity = 0.6 m s^{-1} and f_T = 5 MHz, then using θ_{mid} the scanner would calculate the velocity as being 0.77 m s^{-1}.

If we wish to calculate the average velocity of blood in the sample volume, the situation is different. Calculating the average velocity depends on knowing the strength of the signals from all the Doppler frequencies and from all Doppler angles seen by the transducer. For this purpose some average angle must be used which is likely to be close to θ_{mid}.

The operator cannot alter the angle used by the scanner to calibrate the velocity scale. It is therefore important to be aware which method your own scanner uses and when necessary to take into account the errors produced. An example of the need to be careful would be when measurements from two scanners, each using a different method, are being compared. One way to overcome the problem would be to use a Doppler Phantom whose velocity was known to produce a set of correction tables that could be applied to measurements made on the scanner.

Wall-thump filter

The wall-thump filter is used to remove high-amplitude low-frequency Doppler shifts caused by specular reflection from the slowly moving vessel wall (Figure 1.1). Movement of the wall produces Doppler frequencies close to the heart rate, so the wall-thump filter is typically set to cut out frequencies at < 150 Hz. As some of the true spectral information on flow is removed by the filter, there will be some error in the average velocity calculation (Figure 2.20). The wall-thump filter should always be set to a minimum frequency compatible with its purpose of eliminating unwanted wall echoes.

Clinical note
Vessel measurements and Doppler mode

To make a measurement of the vessel on the B-mode image, for example vessel diameter, the vessel should be imaged so that the vessel walls are at 90° to the direction of propagation of the ultrasound beam. They will then give the sharpest image and errors in the measurement will be minimised. On the other hand, the recording of a good-quality Doppler waveform requires a beam-to-vessel angle of ≤60°. The recording of waveforms and making of B-mode measurements should therefore be performed using the correct angle of approach for each and not combined from a single compromised angle of approach.

Colour-flow imaging

In colour-flow imaging (CFI), also known as colour Doppler ultrasound (CDU), a colour display is superimposed on the normal B-mode image to show areas within the image where echoes are Doppler shifted. This will show flow in blood vessels and within cavities such as in the chambers of the heart and in false aneurysms. The colour map consists of a series of image lines each divided into pixels (Figure 2.21).

Each pixel is filled with a colour whose hue or saturation is proportional to the *mean* Doppler frequency of the echoes from the pixel sample volume. Most scanners allow a choice of colour velocity maps to be made. A colour velocity map that changes the hue with increasing mean velocity is probably the easiest to use because the eye is more sensitive to changes in hue than to changes in the saturation of a single colour. Such a map will also indicate the difference between the maximum velocities both towards and away from the transducer as two different colours, for example yellow and green (Figure 2.22).

Note that a change of hue will occur with:

- Change in velocity, for example due to normal change in vessel calibre or due to stenosis.

- Change in vessel angle with respect to the transducer.

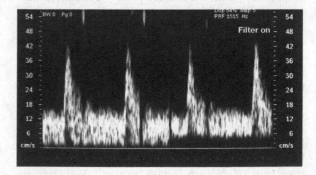

Figure 2.20 – Waveform with the wall-thump filter set too high showing a loss of low Doppler frequencies.

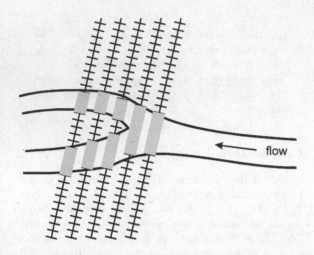

Figure 2.21 – Creation of a colour-flow image by dividing colour-imaging lines into pixels and colouring them in where flow is detected.

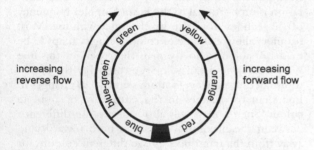

Figure 2.22 – Changes in hue used in colour-flow imaging to render forward and reverse mean Doppler frequency. Adjacent colours passing through black indicate a change in direction; passing from yellow to green, or vice versa, indicates aliasing due to high velocities.

In pixels where the flow is 90° to the transducer, no colour will be shown and the pixel will then typically appear black. Different colours show direction of flow towards or away from the transducer, e.g. red and blue. A change in colour on the display from one direction to the other, passing through black, indicates a change in direction of flow relative to the transducer. As with the Doppler spectrum, the CFI information is sampled over a number of pulses. Therefore the CFI frequency shifts may be under-sampled by the ultrasound system and aliasing will occur. This appears as high-velocity flow in one direction appearing as high-velocity flow in the opposite direction and the spectrum of colours 'wraps around'. A change in colour on the display from one direction to the other, passing through the high-velocity hues, is aliasing and

indicates velocities above the set scale. This aliasing effect may be used to advantage to show regions of high velocity as, for example, in flow through a stenosis or a cardiac jet.

Clinical note
Colour-flow imaging and frame rate

To obtain an adequate estimate of the mean Doppler frequency the scanner must send eight to twelve pulses for each colour line. This has significant implications for the frame rate as the scanner has to share time between producing the CFI display and the B-mode image. The number of pulses per line may be determined by the operator on some scanners as a colour quality control. The fewer the number of pulses the more colour speckle will be seen within an area of flow as the Doppler frequency estimate will be poorer. Generally, the colour display will have a lower line density and therefore be of poorer resolution than the B-mode display in order to maintain frame rate. The operator can improve the frame rate by reducing the region on the image over which the colour information is displayed. Fewer colour lines are then required and more time is available to update the image. It is particularly important to use a small 'colour box' over the region of interest when viewing rapidly moving structures such as the heart. When viewing blood vessels, a high frame rate and the detection of rapid movement is not so important. The use of a large colour box can then be used to give an overall view of where flow is present and to highlight any areas of interest, such as stenoses, for further investigation.

Role of colour-flow imaging in a haemodynamic investigation

The CFI display is used:

- To give a picture of the overall pattern of flow within the B-mode image.

- To indicate the direction of flow.

- To demonstrate vessel patency.

- To highlight regions of interest such as jets, stenoses, etc. that warrant closer study. The spectral Doppler sample volume may then be placed over the region of interest to obtain a Doppler waveform.

- To show up vessels that are not resolvable on the B-mode image, for instance in arteriovenous malformations. The vessels may be too small to be seen on the B-mode image, but if there is flow, a Doppler signal will be detected and the vessel coloured in on the CFI display.

- To indicate the contour of an atheromatous plaque, for example in the presence of plaque ulceration or when the plaque is of very low echogenicity.

The CFI display should not generally be used to make quantitative measurements:

- It is inappropriate to make velocity measurements from the CFI display. This is because, first, the colour/pixel value is proportional to mean velocity not peak velocity. Peak values are diagnostically more useful. Second, the Doppler angle is not usually known. Many scanners show a velocity alongside the colour scale. This velocity assumes that Doppler angle is zero degrees, which is rarely the true Doppler angle. To make reliable velocity measurements, the Doppler waveform from the site of interest should be obtained. The angle cursor should be correctly aligned and measurements should be made from the waveform.

- Significant errors may be made in measuring vessel diameters from the width of flow as indicated by the colour display. The signal processing used to produce the colour display must distinguish between stationary and moving targets. There is a cut-off point, similar to the spectral Doppler wall-thump filter, below which the B-mode image is shown without any colour. This means that either the colour will not always fill the whole vessel lumen to the vessel wall or that the colour will spill over the edge because of echoes arising from a moving wall. Both of these cases will lead to inaccurate measurements of the vessel lumen. To make a reliable direct measurement of vessel calibre use the B-mode image. Image the vessel in longitudinal section at 90° to the direction of propagation of the ultrasound beam when the surfaces of the vessel wall will then be seen most clearly. Use the measurement callipers to measure the vessel lumen. However, it is not always possible to make a measurement from the B-mode image in this way. An estimate of lumen diameter may then be made from the CFI display recognising the possible errors involved. In the case of generalised narrowing, the width of the lumen as shown by CFI allows a qualitative estimate of the severity of narrowing to be made. CFI is also useful in cardiac work for estimating the severity of valve regurgitation and septal defects from the width and length of the flow jet. The degree of colour filling on the image may be controlled by the operator using the colour priority control available on some scanners. This determines the signal strength at which the displaying colour is given priority over the display of the B-mode grey levels.

Clinical note
Checking for vessel patency

To establish whether there is any residual patency in a possibly occluded vessel:

- Reduce the CFI scale to a very low value. This will display low velocities more clearly and is more sensitive in detecting small targets such as very narrow lumens.

- Increase the CFI gain until the display shows colour 'noise'. Then back-off the gain until the noise just disappears.

- The vessel of interest should be examined using CFI in both longitudinal and transverse sections. Ensure that a Doppler angle is maintained between the transducer and the vessel (Figure 1.3).

- Even if no colour filling is seen, position the pulsed-Doppler sample volume over the vessel and obtain a Doppler spectrum. Do this using both longitudinal and transverse views, when the vessel may be more easily identified and isolated by the sample volume. Use a low-velocity scale setting for the Doppler spectrum.

If none of these procedures shows any flow, the vessel is probably occluded.

Power Doppler

In power Doppler mode a colour display is superimposed on the normal B-mode image in a similar way to CFI, but the colour used is proportional to the total backscattered power in the Doppler signal for each pixel. The backscattered power does not depend on the direction of flow and so the power Doppler display does not show direction of flow, just where flow is. It is less sensitive to Doppler angle and so flows over a wide range of angles may be displayed more easily than with CFI, for example tortuous vessels, kidney parenchyma and flow around a plaque.

Further reading

Evens DH, McDicken WA. *Doppler Ultrasound: Physics, Instrumentation and Clinical Applications*, 2nd edn. Chichester: Wiley, 2000.

3

BASIC HAEMODYNAMICS

BASIC HAEMODYNAMICS

Outline

Basic fluid properties are defined. Phenomena associated with continuous flow in a tube are described including velocity profile and turbulence. Flow through a stenosis and at a bifurcation are examined as are vessel diameter and the mechanics of venous valves.

When observing Doppler waveforms it is important to continually form an answer to the question 'Why does that waveform have the particular shape I see?' because only when we understand why it has that shape and form can we really attempt to say what is going on in the vessels being examined. For example, there are two basic patterns seen in Doppler waveforms obtained from normal arteries (Figure 3.1).

For the purposes of description, Doppler arterial waveforms are divided into two phases related to the cardiac cycle: the **systolic phase**, with a large increase in flow due to the cardiac ventricles contracting and expelling blood into the circulation, and a **diastolic phase**, occurring when the aortic valve has closed and the ventricles are refilling. In one waveform type, seen in the aorta and long arteries of the limbs, there is little or no flow during diastole (Figure 3.1a). There may even be some reverse flow as shown. In the second waveform type (Figure 3.1b), seen in arteries supplying organs such as the brain, placenta or kidneys, there is forward flow throughout diastole. The distribution of grey levels within the Doppler spectrum varies between the two phases and the overall shape of the waveform will vary from one artery to another. Why do these two types differ so much? **Haemodynamics** is the physics of blood flow and it provides a physical explanation of the waveforms seen. Armed with that information a more confident and reliable report of the findings of a vascular ultrasound investigation may be given.

Fluid properties

There are two fundamental properties of a fluid that are important when determining fluid motion: density and viscosity.

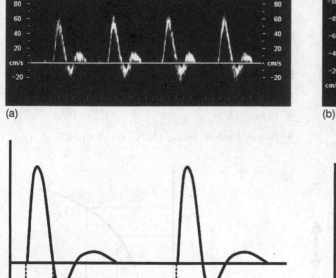

(a)

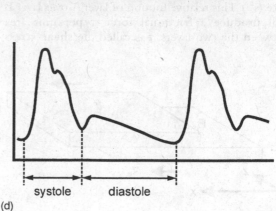

(b)

(c)

(d)

Figure 3.1 – The two basic waveform shapes showing the systolic and diastolic phases of each.

Density

Density (ρ) (kgm^{-3})

Density is the mass per unit volume of the fluid. A fluid such as blood is usually considered incompressible and so its density is constant. Any small variation in density with temperature may be neglected over a 0–50°C range and in the flow conditions seen in the circulation.

Examples:

- Water (21°C): 998 kg m^{-3}
- Plasma (37°C): 1027 kg m^{-3}
- Whole blood (37°C): 1060 kg m^{-3}

Viscosity

Viscosity (μ) (kg m^{-1} s^{-1} = Pa s (Pascal seconds))

Colloquially speaking, viscosity is a measure of the 'syrupiness' of a fluid, i.e. how thick it is. It determines how easy it is to move an object such as a spoon through the fluid or how easily it will flow along a pipe. For example, water has a low viscosity compared with syrup. Viscosity is caused by the internal frictional forces within the fluid as the molecules of the fluid move past one another. Consider one thin layer of a fluid A moving more quickly over an adjacent layer B in the x-direction (Figure 3.2).

This sliding of one microscopic layer over another is known as **shear**. The velocity of the fluid is increasing in the y-direction as shown in Figure 3.2b. Thus, layer A moves over layer B with the velocity difference $\Delta v = v_A - v_B$. The velocity gradient in the y-direction is therefore $\Delta v/\Delta y$ and is called the **shear rate** (s^{-1}). This relative motion of layer A over layer B will produce a frictional force τ per unit area between the two layers. τ is called the **shear stress**

(N m^{-2} = Pa). This force will act so as to accelerate the slower moving layer and drag on the faster moving layer. The relationship between the shear stress and the velocity gradient is given by:

$$\tau = \mu \frac{\Delta v}{\Delta y}, \text{(kg m}^{-1}\text{ s}^{-2} = \text{N m}^{-2})$$

where μ is the **coefficient of viscosity** or just the viscosity. If the viscosity in a fluid is constant for all velocity changes, or shear rates, it is known as a **Newtonian fluid**. In the large vessels of the body, blood effectively behaves as a Newtonian fluid. However, at very low shear rates and in vessels < 1 mm diameter, the behaviour is non-Newtonian and the viscosity varies with the velocity gradient. At very low shear rates viscosity increases and in small sub-millimetre vessels the viscosity of blood actually decreases. These effects occur because blood is a complex fluid containing particles in suspension in plasma containing long molecules of fibrinogen. In low shear conditions rouleaux formation by RBC causes viscosity to increase.

The viscosity of blood also depends on temperature and haematocrit. For whole blood there is about a 51% increase in viscosity on decreasing temperature from 37 to 25°C. Change in viscosity with haematocrit is shown in Figure 3.3 for two shear rates.

These changes in viscosity can have important consequences for flow and the work done by the heart in pathological conditions such as hypothermia, polycythaemia and severe anaemia.

Examples:

- Water (21°C): 1 m Pa s
- Plasma (37°C): 1.2 m Pa s
- Normal whole blood (37°C): ~4 m Pa s

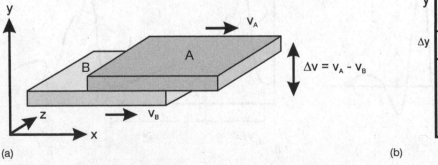
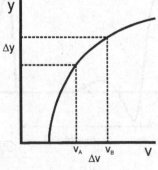

Figure 3.2 – Diagram showing two fluid layers A and B moving with respect to one another illustrating the definition of shear rate.

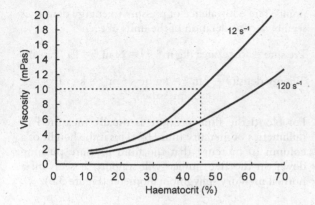

Figure 3.3 – Graph of viscosity against haematocrit for whole human blood at 37° shown for two shear rates. Broken line indicates normal haematocrit.[14]

Volume flow

The volume of blood flowing through an artery is of fundamental importance as it is the volume flow that determines the oxygen carried by the vessel. To calculate the volume flow when the velocity across the vessel lumen may not be constant and the velocity is also changing with time over the cardiac cycle, the mean velocity $\bar{v}$ must be used. This is also known as the **time average velocity** (TAV).

In Figure 3.4, using the velocity equation $v = s/t$, where v is velocity, s is distance and t is time, the surface A will move through a distance $\bar{v}$ in 1 s. The volume of the shaded cylinder Q within the vessel lumen will then be:

$$Q = A.\bar{v} \ \ (m^3 \ s^{-1})$$

Volume Flow Equation

This is called the volume flow equation. If a circular cross-section is assumed, the cross-sectional area may be calculated from the vessel diameter D using:

$$A = \frac{\pi D^2}{4} = \pi r^2$$

Figure 3.4 – Diagram defining the volume flow equation.

It is common to measure volume flow in millilitres per minute (ml min^{-1}). If the linear measurements are measured in centimetres and the result multiplied by 60, flow in millilitres per minute is obtained.

Clinical note
Measuring volume flow

Most duplex scanners allow TAV to be calculated from the Doppler waveform. Volume flow may then be found by measuring TAV over a complete number of cardiac cycles and multiplying TAV with the cross-sectional area calculated from the vessel diameter. In practice the calculation of volume flow is subject to large systematic and random errors that are not easily overcome. They result from factors such as non-uniform insonation of the vessel by narrow, highly focussed ultrasound beams, changes in vessel diameter over the cardiac cycle and measurement inaccuracies. For example, any error in measuring the diameter will be squared in the area calculation. Errors can be minimised by choosing a wide, straight vessel and by using a wide-range gate that straddles the vessel. Make the diameter measurement from the same point on the vessel that the Doppler spectrum is obtained. Then make several measurements of both the diameter and TAV and take the mean of each to reduce the random measurement errors. Useful estimates of cardiac output and flow through arteriovenous fistulae in the brachial artery of dialysis patients may be made, but the error associated with the estimates is still likely to be of the order $\pm 12\%$.[2]

In a tube with no branches, the volume flow must be constant throughout its length, and at bifurcations the sum of the flow in the branches must equal the flow in the parent vessel. This is equivalent to saying that mass is conserved in the flow. It is expressed in the **continuity equation**, which is used to assess the degree of stenosis in heart valves (Figure 3.5).

$$A_2 = A_1 \frac{\bar{v}_1}{\bar{v}_2}$$

The same flow passes both points and since the area A_2 is smaller, the velocity $\bar{v}_2$ must be larger. This is the same effect as seen in a river flowing more swiftly through a

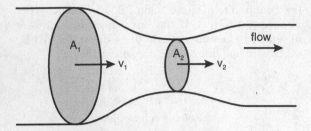

Figure 3.5 – Diagram defining the continuity equation.

narrow gorge than along a wide stretch. Assuming that the highest velocity occurs at the valve orifice, an estimate of the valve cross-sectional area can be made from measurements of the outflow tract area A_1 and the mean velocities at the two locations.

Energy density

The movement of blood round the circulation requires energy. The way in which energy changes form and is lost around the system has a direct effect on blood flow and hence the Doppler waveforms seen. The total energy associated with blood flow consists of two components: **potential energy** and **kinetic energy**.

Potential energy is stored energy from which the kinetic energy associated with the movement of blood is derived:

$$E_{total} = \text{potential energy} + \text{kinetic energy} \quad (\text{joule}, J)$$

Unlike a solid, rigid object, a fluid such as blood is a continuum of lightly bound microscopic particles of fixed volume that will tend to move to fill any container it is in, changing shape as it does so. For this reason we consider energy density rather than energy itself. This is the energy associated with a particular volume of fluid regardless of its shape:

$$\text{Energy density} = \text{energy/volume} \quad (Jm^{-3})$$

Blood pressure

For a fluid the potential energy is equal to the pressure of the fluid on an object placed within it. This is known as **fluid pressure** or, in the case of blood, **blood pressure**. At any particular location in a fluid at rest, the pressure is the same in all directions. Also, because the fluid is incompressible, a change in pressure at one point will be transmitted through the fluid to all other points. The equivalence of pressure to energy density is seen by a consideration of the units of each:

Pressure = force/area ($kg\ m^{-1}\ s^{-2} = N\ m^{-2} = Pa$ (Pascal))

Energy density = $J\ m^{-3} = kg\ m^2\ s^{-2}\ m^{-3} = kg\ m^{-1}\ s^{-2} =$ pressure

For blood the fluid pressure is usually measured in millimetres of mercury (mmHg). This is the height of a column of mercury that the fluid pressure pushing down on the free surface will support, as seen on a normal mercury sphygmomanometer (Figure 3.6).

Conversion factor: 1 mmHg = 133.3 Pa

There are three components to fluid pressure in the circulation. These must be added together to give the total pressure at any point.

● **Static filling pressure** (P_S): residual pressure that exists in a supine person in the absence of any arterial flow, e.g. the blood pressure in a dead person. It results from the fact that the circulation is a closed system and depends on the total blood volume and elastic properties of the vessel walls. It is equivalent to the pressure in a partially blown up bicycle tyre. The static filling pressure is typically 5–10 mmHg.

● **Hydrostatic pressure** (P_{HS}): fluid pressure due to the force of gravity acting between two points. For

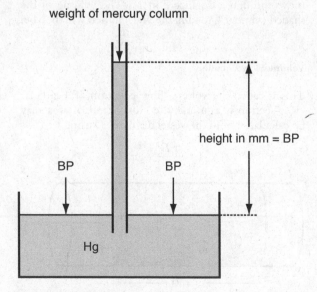

Figure 3.6 – Diagram defining the measurement of blood pressure in millimetres of mercury.

instance, hydrostatic pressure is the pressure felt by a swimmer as they dive deeper into water. It is due to the weight of water above pressing down and so depends on the difference in height (h) between two points and the acceleration due to gravity ($g = 9.81$ m s^{-2}). Hydrostatic pressure has a negative sign because an increase in height produces a drop in pressure:

$$\text{Hydrostatic pressure: } P_{HS} = \rho g h$$

$$P_{HS} = 10398.6 \times h \text{ (Pa)} = 78 \times h \text{ (mmHg)}$$

The zero pressure reference point in the body is taken to be the right atrium of the heart. The actual blood pressure in the right atrium is ~10 mmHg (Table 3.1).

Hydrostatic pressure is a real pressure difference, i.e. it can be measured. However, unlike water flowing down a river where the force of gravity moves the water along,

Table 3.1 – Examples of hydrostatic pressure

Position	Distance (m)		Pressure (mmHg)
Lying supine	head–foot:	1.7	0
Standing	heart–head:	0.4	−40
	heart–foot:	−1.3	+100
Fighter pilot in a 6g turn	heart–head:	0.4	−190
	heart–foot:	−1.0	+470

hydrostatic pressure in the circulation is not available to do work on moving the blood around. This is because the circulation is a closed system. Figure 3.7 shows that the increase in pressure in the foot when standing is exactly balanced by the work required to lift the blood against gravity back to the heart again. Therefore, the fluid remains static if no other force is applied.

Although it is not available to do work and move blood around, hydrostatic pressure and changes in it do have

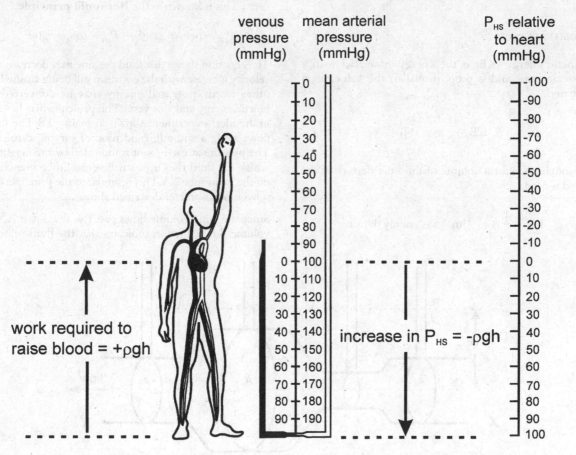

Figure 3.7 – Variation in blood pressure in a standing adult. Values are the sum of mean dynamic pressure and hydrostatic pressure. The increase in hydrostatic pressure towards the feet is seen to equal the work required to lift the blood back to the heart against the force of gravity.

important clinical and physiological consequences. For example, the development of varicose veins is exacerbated by maintaining an upright posture, and the sudden drop in cerebral pressure upon sitting or standing up must be corrected by the body's mechanisms of autoregulation.

- **Dynamic pressure** (P_D): increase in fluid pressure produced by contraction of the ventricles of the heart. It is only this component of the total fluid pressure that is available to do work on the blood, driving it around the circulation. The dynamic pressure produced by the heart normally varies between 70 and 130 mmHg across the cardiac cycle, but systolic pressure may be double this in a person with hypertension.

How much energy is stored as pressure?

Systolic pressure = 120 mmHg × 133.3 = 15 996 Jm^{-3}

KINETIC ENERGY

Kinetic energy (KE) is the energy associated with a moving mass and is proportional to the velocity (v) squared:

$$KE = \frac{1}{2} m v^2 \ (J)$$

To obtain KE for a volume of fluid the density of the fluid is used:

$$KE = \frac{1}{2} \rho v^2 \ (Jm^{-3}) \text{ i.e. energy density}$$

How big is kinetic energy in normal arteries?

$$\rho = 1.06 \times 10^3 \text{ kg m}^{-3}$$

At peak systole: $v = 0.6$ m s^{-1}, then KE = 190 J m^{-3}

Notice that this is very small compared with the potential energy due to the fluid pressure.

Blood flows around the circulation as a result of differences in **total fluid energy**. In particular it flows down a pressure gradient:

$$E_{Tot} = P_S + (-\rho gh) + P_D + (\tfrac{1}{2}\rho v^2) \ (J m^{-3})$$

Just as the mass of the fluid does not change, energy is also conserved as a fluid moves along a vessel. Assuming no energy is lost due to friction and there is steady flow, the total energy equation may be written to show the conservation of energy at two points, X and Y, along the vessel. This is known as the **Bernoulli principle**:

$$P_{DX} - \rho gh_x + \tfrac{1}{2}\rho v^2_x = P_{DY} - \rho gh_y + \tfrac{1}{2}\rho v^2_y$$

The equation shows that fluid pressure may decrease and velocity increase with the equation still being satisfied. In other words, potential energy may be converted to kinetic energy and vice versa. This principle may be seen in the ideal experiment shown in Figure 3.8. The fluid flows along a smooth, rigid tube of varying diameter. The pressure at each point is indicated by the height to which the fluid rises up a small vertical tube branching off the main tube XY. This is similar to the principle of a sphygmomanometer described above.

Since the same volume flows past Y as flows past X, the volume flow equation indicates that the fluid velocity

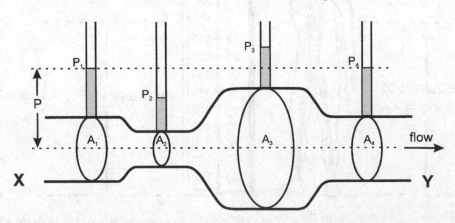

Figure 3.8 – Illustration of the Bernoulli principle.

will be higher at A_2 than at A_1, and will be lower at A_3 than at A_1. The Bernoulli principle indicates that in order for energy to be conserved, the increase in velocity at A_2 must be accompanied by a corresponding decrease in fluid pressure. This is seen in the reduced height to which the fluid rises up the vertical tube P_2 relative to P_1. Similarly at A_3 the velocity is lower and kinetic energy is transferred into potential energy and the fluid pressure rises above P_1.

In a real vessel, energy will in fact be lost in the form of heat due to friction experienced by the moving fluid. Some of the energy transferring from potential energy to kinetic energy in the accelerating and decelerating blood will also be lost along the way in the form of heat. In practice this means that while we see a drop in fluid pressure accompanying a rise in velocity, less kinetic energy is returned to potential energy as velocity drops. As a result, there is an overall drop in fluid pressure as blood moves around the circulation. The **mean dynamic pressure** averaged over the cardiac cycle will always get lower as the blood moves towards the periphery of the arterial tree.

PRESSURE HALF-TIME – FOR THE MITRAL VALVE

Looking at the Bernoulli principle and the volume flow equation, a method for estimating valve area is suggested that has proved useful when examining the mitral valve. The valve separates two elastic chambers with pressures P_1 and P_2 where, at the start of diastole, $P_1 > P_2$ (Figure 3.9). The assumption is made from the Bernoulli principle that pressure P_1 is converted into moving the blood through the valve at a velocity proportional to v^2. As pressure P_1 drops, the velocity through the valve will also fall and the rate of drop in pressure can be found by timing the fall in velocity. Since, when pressure is converted to velocity, the pressure drop is proportional to velocity squared, the time taken for the velocity to fall to $\sqrt{2}$ of its initial value is measured to find when the

pressure has halved. This is known as the **pressure half-time** (PHT) and is measured in milliseconds (ms). Measurement is made over the first part of the slope when the pressure difference between the two chambers is greatest (Figure 3.10).

The rate at which the velocity falls will depend on the cross-sectional area of the valve and hence the flow through it. However, the absolute value of velocity will depend on the pressure difference $P_1 - P_2$, which will be affected by heart rate and regurgitation across the

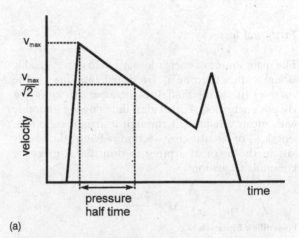

(a)

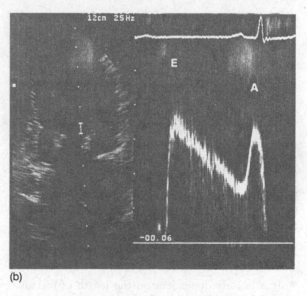

(b)

Figure 3.10 – a) Diagrammatic representation of the waveform seen in the mitral valve during diastole, illustrating the measurement of the pressure half time. b) the Doppler waveform. Note, the first peak occurs as passive filling of the ventricle takes place, the second peak occurs during atrial contraction.

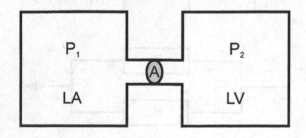

Figure 3.9 – Diagram defining the pressures in the left atrium and left ventricle of the heart during diastole.

valve when it is closed. The relationship between pressure half-time and cross-sectional area of the valve has been derived empirically by measurement of post-mortem specimens. This has produced the relationship:

$$220/\text{PHT} = \text{mitral valve area (cm}^2).$$

PHT < 60 ms is seen in normal valves, with 100–400 ms or higher indicating stenosis. Measurement of valve area by this method is independent of heart rate and valve regurgitation.

Frictional losses

The main source of energy loss as a fluid moves steadily along a smooth tube is frictional loss due to the viscosity (μ) of the fluid. It is therefore also known as viscous energy loss. For an ideal fluid flowing smoothly with mean velocity ($\bar{v}$) through a straight rigid tube length (l) of circular cross-section radius (r) the energy loss in the form of a pressure drop ΔP is given by Poiseuille's equation:

$$\Delta P = \frac{\bar{v}8l\mu}{r^2}$$

Poiseuille's Equation

Using the volume flow equation to substitute for velocity in Poiseuille's equation:

$$Q = A.v = \pi r^2 v$$

$$\Delta P = Q \cdot \left(\frac{8l\mu}{\pi r^4}\right) = Q \cdot R_f$$

where Q is volume flow and R_f is **fluid resistance**. Note that Poiseuille's equation is the fluid equivalent of Ohm's law of electrical resistance (Table 3.2).

Poiseuille's equation is a measure of the work that must be done to move the fluid along a tube of length l. Note the following points:

- It is very strongly dependent on the radius of the tube, to the fourth power.
- It is linearly dependent on the length of the tube and the viscosity of the fluid.
- It is linearly dependent on the velocity of the fluid.

We shall see that these factors have important consequences for blood flow in diseased arteries.

Table 3.2 – Ohm's law and Poiseuille's equation compared

	Ohm's law: $V = I\,R$	Poiseuille's equation: $\Delta P = Q\,R_f$
Driving force	voltage difference	pressure difference
Current	electric current	volume flow
Resistance	electrical resistance	fluid resistance

Peripheral vascular resistance

Every artery is a fluid resistor as given by Poiseuille's equation. The resistance of the normal large arteries is relatively small producing a pressure drop of <5 mmHg Figure 6.1. The effective resistance in diseased arteries can be very much higher. Most of the pressure drop in the normal circulation occurs at the arteriole–capillary level, but the larger arteries will 'see' a resistance into which blood flows. Peripheral vascular resistance describes the total resistance seen by an artery distal to the point of observation. Where there are several resistances along the vessel, they may be considered together by adding them as for electrical resistance (Figure 3.11):

Examples of resistances in series are multiple stenoses in a vessel segment and a vessel segment followed by end organ resistance. Examples of resistances in parallel are the branches of a bifurcation and flow to an end organ via collateral routes.

$$\text{(a)} \quad R_T = R_1 + R_2$$

$$\text{(b)} \quad \frac{1}{R_T} = \frac{1}{R_1} + \frac{1}{R_2}$$

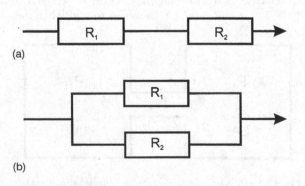

(a)

(b)

Figure 3.11 – Resistors in a) series and b) parallel circuit.

Diastolic flow

In arteries that have waveforms with a continuous forward component of flow throughout the cardiac cycle (Figure 3.1b), flow during the diastolic phase is very dependent upon the peripheral resistance that the artery sees. If the pressure drop across the peripheral resistance is greater than diastolic pressure, then there will be no flow during diastole. If it is less than diastolic pressure, flow will depend on the residual pressure difference. Flow during systole is much greater than during diastole as the residual pressure difference is much greater and it is not so significantly altered by changes in peripheral resistance. For this reason, the flow in diastole is a good indicator of whether the normal end organ is a high- or low-resistance circuit. Changes in diastolic flow from expected values can indicate pathological changes in the end organ or distal disease in the artery itself (Table 3.3).

Paradoxically, continuous flow in diastole may be seen in a vessel normally having a zero end-diastolic flow when there is distal disease in the vessel. It occurs when the distal disease restricts the outflow causing the pressure gradient across the diseased segment to remain positive throughout the cardiac cycle. There is then forward flow throughout the cycle. An example of this is the presence of a long third component in the waveform of the femoral artery (Figure 3.12). This waveform usually indicates a distal stenosis or generalised narrowing distally.

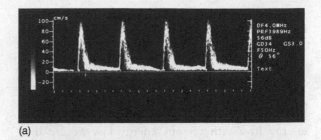

(a)

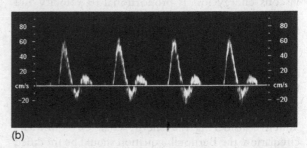

(b)

Figure 3.12 – Doppler waveform obtained from common femoral artery in a patient with severe superficial femoral disease. (a) Note the long third component extending throughout diastole. b) Normal triphasic waveform shown for comparison.

INERTIA FORCES

If a fluid is made to move in a particular direction by forces such as a pressure gradient or friction, the fluid will tend to resist that acceleration in proportion to its mass. This resisting force F is known as inertia force and is given by Newton's second law, which states that

$$\text{Force} = \text{mass} \times \text{acceleration}$$

which for a fluid volume l^3 of density ρ with change in velocity Δv in time t, the inertia force is:

$$F = \rho l^3 \cdot \frac{\Delta v}{t} \ (\text{kg m s}^{-2} = \text{N})$$

Inertial energy losses

Just as friction results in energy loss to the flow as given by Poiseuille's equation, so there will be situations where inertia forces result in energy losses to the system. Inertial energy losses may occur whenever there is a change in direction of flow or a change in velocity. This is because it requires work to be done on the mass of fluid to bring about these changes and some of this energy will be lost to the circulation.

Table 3.3 – Examples of high, low and variable resistance flows

Resistance flow	Normal diastolic flow	Abnormal changes
High	External carotid to face and neck.	Reduced flow to transplanted liver/kidney.
Low	internal carotid to brain; renal flow.	Arteriovenous malformation.
Variable	Flow to the hand changes with temperature; mesenteric flow – eating/fasting; placental flow – age of gestation.	Raynaud's phenomenon – abnormal response to temperature in the extremities.

Inertial energy losses ΔE involve terms similar to the kinetic energy term in the Bernoulli equation, i.e.

$$\Delta E = k \; \tfrac{1}{2}\rho\Delta v^2$$

where ρ is fluid density, Δv is velocity change and k is a constant giving the proportion of energy which is lost, due to a change in velocity. Comparing this energy loss with viscous energy loss we see that viscous energy loss is proportional to velocity and inertial energy loss is proportional to velocity squared. In terms of magnitude, losses due to inertial effects are very low in normal vessels, but because of the v^2 term they may increase to exceed viscous energy losses. This is especially likely in the presence of disease where the lumen of an artery is rapidly changing in diameter and flow becomes turbulent.

When considering the energy changes around the circulation, the Bernoulli equation should be modified to include these energy losses:

$$P_{DX} - \rho g h_X + \tfrac{1}{2}\rho v_X^2 = P_{DY} - \rho g h_Y + \tfrac{1}{2}\rho v_Y^2 - \Delta P_{poiseuille} - \Delta E_{inertial}$$

Before we consider flow through a stenosis, we look at the way flow changes as flow velocity increases.

Streamlines

To show the way fluid flows down a tube, a diagram can be drawn showing the paths taken by individual particles of fluid within the flow (Figure 3.13). The path that one particle takes within the mass of fluid is called a streamline.

Where the tube gets narrower the streamlines are pushed together. The flow velocity will also increase, so the spacing between streamlines indicates the speed of

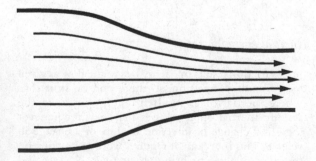

Figure 3.13 – Diagram showing streamlines.

flow. The relative lengths of the streamlines may also show velocity. Streamlines can be made to show up in clear fluids such as water by injecting a small amount of dye from a tiny nozzle into the moving fluid. The path of the dye downstream from the nozzle will show the streamline. Flow through glass models of arteries has been studied using this technique (Figure 3.43).

Velocity profile

In general, fluid velocity will vary across the diameter of a vessel. Intuitively we may expect it to be slow near the stationary vessel walls due to friction with the walls and faster at the centre of the vessel. Flow in the middle of a river is usually faster than at the edges. When fluid is flowing smoothly in layers, with no mixing of fluid between layers, the flow is said to be **laminar**. In this situation all motion in the fluid is parallel to the vessel walls, i.e. parallel streamlines, with no radial components of velocity.

PARABOLIC FLOW

In a smooth, rigid tube with slow continuous flow, the layer of fluid next to the stationary tube wall is slowed by friction with the wall. Immediately adjacent to the wall the fluid velocity is zero. The layer of fluid next to the first layer will move more easily but will still be slowed by friction with that first, slowly moving layer. This description may be continued to all further layers. Moving away from the wall, the velocity in each successive layer is then a bit faster than in the previous layer. The result is shown in Figure 3.14a, where each layer is shown as a concentric annulus within the tube, with the fastest flow occurring along the centre line of tube. In reality, each 'layer' is infinitesimally thin and the velocity profile that develops is shown in Figure 3.14b.

The shape of the velocity profile $v(r)$ as the radius r increases to the full vessel radius R, and v_{max} is the centre line velocity is given by:

$$v(r) = \left(1 - \frac{r^2}{R^2}\right)v_{max}$$

This is the formula of a parabola, and so this type of laminar flow is also known as **parabolic flow**. It has the property that the volume of fluid moving at each velocity (i.e. the volume of each annulus) up to v_{max} is constant. Therefore for blood, the number of RBC moving at each velocity will be constant (k) (Figure 3.15a).

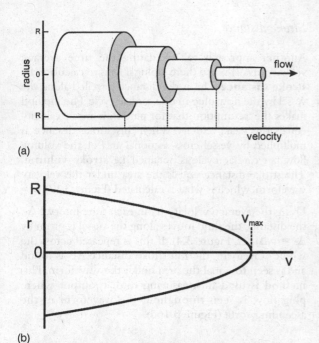

(a)

(b)

Figure 3.14 – Parabolic velocity profile shown a) as a series of concentric laminae and b) as a continuous curve of infinitesimally thin laminae.

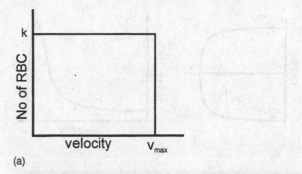

(a)

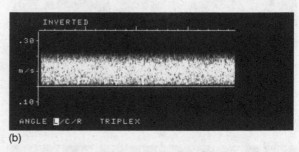

(b)

Figure 3.15 – Spectrum of velocities produced by a parabolic velocity profile a) in terms of amount of blood moving at each velocity and b) as seen on a Doppler spectrum.

For blood flowing with a parabolic profile, with uniform insonation across the whole vessel, the Doppler spectrum will have the same grey level for all velocities up to v_{max} (Figure 3.15b). Examples of a spectrum showing a parabolic velocity profile are those seen in veins and the diastolic phase of some arterial flows.

Note: it is a property of a parabolic velocity profile that the mean velocity $\bar{v}$ is equal to half the maximum velocity v_{max}

$$\bar{v} = \frac{v_{max}}{2}$$

This fact has been used to estimate mean velocity by measuring the peak velocity envelope and dividing by two. It is only valid when the velocity profile is truly parabolic in shape.

PLUG FLOW

As flow in the tube increases the velocity profile becomes flatter (Figure 3.16a). The velocity at the tube wall is still zero, but velocity increases more rapidly away from the wall, i.e. there is a higher shear rate. Nearly all the fluid across the lumen then moves within a narrow range of high velocities. It is as though all the fluid layers across the lumen of the tube were moving along together as a solid plug. For this reason, this type of flow is known as **plug flow**.

Figure 3.16b shows the number of RBC moving at each velocity for plug flow. The Doppler spectrum will have a high grey level over a narrow range of high velocities with much lower grey levels below this range as shown. An example of a spectrum showing a plug flow-velocity profile is that seen at the systolic peak of an arterial waveform. This gives the characteristic 'window' seen under the systolic peak. Where there is plug flow, with the velocities occurring over a very narrow range, the mean velocity will be very close to the maximum velocity. In this situation an estimate of the time average velocity may be made using the average value of the peak velocity envelope and taking that as equal to the mean velocity.

The change in velocity profile that is seen at various points within the Doppler waveform from an artery is complicated by the fact that the velocity of blood is pulsatile and changes over the cardiac cycle.

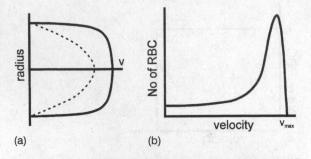

(a)　　　　　　　　　　　(b)

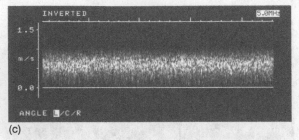

(c)

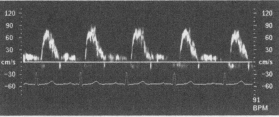

(d) Systolic 'window'

Figure 3.16 – 'Plug flow' velocity profile shown a) as a velocity profile (solid line) with a parabolic profile (broken line) shown for comparison. b) in terms of amount of blood moving at each velocity and c) as seen on a Doppler spectrum. d) Shows the 'window' under the systolic peak in a waveform from ascending aorta.

Stroke distance

Another approach to calculating the time average velocity (TAV) when there is plug flow is to calculate the **stroke distance**. This is the distance travelled along the vessel by the flow plug in one cardiac cycle. The method makes the assumption that for plug flow mean velocity equals the peak velocity. When this stroke distance is multiplied by vessel cross-sectional area A, the volume flow per cardiac cycle is obtained, i.e. **stroke volume**. The stroke distance equals the area under the velocity waveform, which is what is calculated (Figure 3.17).

Using the average velocity (v) in each time interval Δt, the distance the fluid moves along the vessel is given by $\Delta s = v.\Delta t$ (cf. Figure 3.4). If this is repeated across the whole waveform, the full stroke distance AB is found and is seen to equal the area under the waveform. This method is used in measuring cardiac output where plug flow is seen throughout the waveform in the ascending aorta (Figure 3.16d).

Clinical note
Measuring cardiac output

The cross-sectional area A of the aortic root is calculated from a diameter measurement, for example, from an M-mode trace. The velocity waveform is then obtained by viewing the aortic root along the axis of the ascending aorta from the suprasternal notch. From this view-point the Doppler angle is zero so cos (θ) = 1. Using pulsed-Doppler, velocities at the aortic root are found by locating the aortic valve,

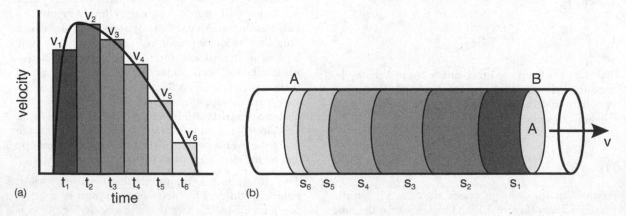

Figure 3.17 – Diagram showing derivation of stroke distance (b) as area under systolic peak of the Doppler spectrum (a).

recognised by audible clicks of the leaflets moving, and then reducing the sample volume depth slightly to bring it into the aortic root. Because plug flow is seen and a single valued velocity waveform can be assumed, the time average velocity is equal to the stroke distance SD multiplied by the heart rate HR. The volume flow equation then becomes:

$$CO = SD \times HR \times A$$

and stroke distance is found by measuring the area under the systolic peak of the velocity waveform.

Turbulence and Reynolds number

From an examination of Poiseuille's equation it looks as though we can increase flow in a tube by increasing the pressure gradient, and that we could go on doing that indefinitely. If an experiment is performed and flow in a tube is measured as the driving pressure is increased, a graph of the sort shown in Figure 3.18 is obtained.

At first there is a linear relationship between flow and pressure drop along the tube, as expected from Poiseuille's equation. Over this region flow is laminar with no mixing of streamlines. A point is then reached where the flow increases more slowly in response to

increasing the driving pressure. What is happening is that beyond P_t, turbulence is developing in the fluid. In addition to the energy lost due to viscous friction in laminar flow, energy is being diverted from the bulk flow down the tube into many small, complex eddies and motions. This mixes up all the smooth layers that existed in the laminar flow regime and dissipates energy as heat (Figure 3.19). This is inertial energy loss.

At low flows the viscous forces tend to damp out any tendency for the fluid particles to move 'out of line' and the laminae remain unmixed. At high velocities the fluid particles have enough momentum to move out of their layers to disturb adjacent layers until fully developed turbulence is seen. Reynolds found that the point at which this transition occurred could be determined by looking at the ratio of inertia force to viscous force expressed as a dimensionless number now known as the **Reynolds number** (Re). For a tube diameter D with fluid density ρ, viscosity μ and velocity v, it is given by:

$$Re = \frac{D\rho v}{\mu}$$

Reynold's Number

The Reynolds number is dimensionless, all units cancel.

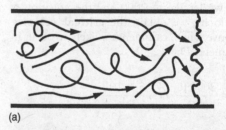

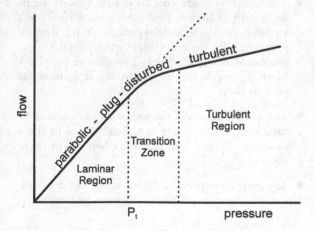

Figure 3.18 – Diagrammatic representation of the pressure–flow curve showing the velocity profiles and flow conditions as pressure and flow increase.

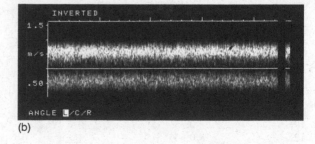

Figure 3.19 – Turbulent flow showing a) streamlines and velocity profile and b) the Doppler spectrum.

Note
Derivation of Reynolds number

For flow in a tube, energy loss due to friction is given by Poiseuille's equation:

$$\Delta P = \frac{\bar{v}8l\mu}{r^2} = \frac{force}{area}$$

therefore, dimensionally, friction force $\propto v l \mu$

Inertia force $F = \rho l^3 . \frac{v}{t} \equiv \rho l^2 v^2$ i

the ratio of these forces is

$$\frac{inertia\ force}{friction\ force} \approx \frac{\rho l^2 v^2}{v l \mu} = \frac{\rho l v}{\mu}$$

If we let length l that characterises the tube be the tube diameter D we have Reynolds number:

$$\mathrm{Re} = \frac{D\rho v}{\mu}$$

for which values can be determined experimentally.

For continuous fluid flow in a straight rigid tube, the transition to turbulent flow occurs between $\mathrm{Re} = 2000$ and 2500. If we let $\mathrm{Re} = 2000$ and the equation is solved for velocity, we obtain the **critical velocity** (Table 3.4) above which turbulence is likely to occur in a vessel of diameter D:

$$v_c = \frac{2000.\mu}{\rho.D} = \frac{7.55 \times 10^{-3}}{D} \ (\mathrm{m\ s^{-1}})$$

Table 3.4 – Critical velocities

Diameter (mm)	Critical velocity (m s⁻¹)
1	7.54
2	3.77
4	1.89
6	1.26
8	0.94
10	0.75
12	0.63
16	0.47
20	0.38

Where there is turbulent flow, the flow is no longer linear with driving pressure and has a power relationship:

$$Q \propto \Delta P^x$$

where x is in the range 0.6–0.5.

This is shown for a 4-mm diameter vessel in Figure 3.20.

Does turbulence occur in the normal circulation?

- Aorta: diameter = 0.026 m, then $v_c = 0.29$ m s⁻¹. At rest PSV in ascending aorta > 0.4 m s⁻¹

- Superficial femoral artery (SFA): diameter = 0.006 m, then $v_c = 1.2$ m s⁻¹. PSV in SFA = 0.8 m s⁻¹

So there may be turbulence in the aortic arch at peak systole. At times of increased cardiac output such as during exercise, turbulence is even more likely to occur there. In more peripheral vessels the critical velocity will be higher because their diameter is smaller and turbulence is less likely. These features are illustrated in Figure 3.21, which assumes continuous flow in straight vessels with no disease present. The line of critical velocity is indicated as is a line showing typical peak systolic velocities in arteries of these diameters.

Note:

- At velocities greater than the critical velocity the flow becomes turbulent and an increase in the pressure drop is seen.

- The velocities lower than the critical velocity are in the region of laminar flow governed by Poiseuille's equation. In this region the pressure drop is directly proportional to the mean velocity, although the linear relation is not immediately obvious (Figure 3.20) from this graph because of the log scale used for pressure drop.

- The smaller the vessel, the higher is v_c. In addition to this, high velocities are not usually seen in small vessels, so flow is almost always laminar in these vessels.

- The increase in pressure drop as vessel size decreases is a consequence of the radius term in Poiseuille's equation.

- Where there is turbulence, the increase in pressure drop shown on this graph is a minimum. Uneven vessel lumen may increase this loss further.

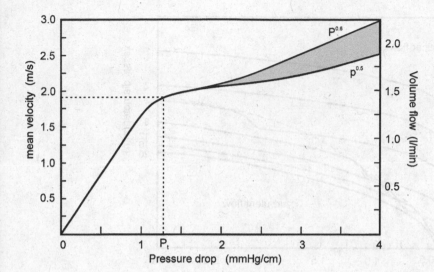

Figure 3.20 – Theoretical pressure–flow curve for blood in a 4mm diameter vessel with steady flow conditions. The range of values when turbulence exists is indicated.

Clinical note
Turbulence in normal vessels

Turbulence may be seen in an otherwise normal vessel when that vessel is acting as collateral for other occluded vessels, e.g. vertebral artery in the presence of common carotid artery-internal carotid artery occlusion. In such a situation, the turbulence is due to large flow. In the absence of disease in the vertebral artery, the vessel's own intrinsic diameter limits flow. The vessel is probably carrying close to its maximal flow. By comparison, flow in the aortic arch may normally be turbulent but any pressure drop is still very small (Figure 3.21).

Once formed, turbulence may propagate downstream as it has a tendency to amplify itself. For example, turbulence seen in both left and right common carotid and subclavian arteries is diagnostic of aortic valve stenosis where it originates. Generally speaking, pulsatile flow is more stable than continuous flow and a higher velocity is required to induce turbulence when flow is pulsatile.

Boundary layer

Adjacent to a vessel wall or any object over which a fluid moves, there will be boundary layer of thickness δ within the fluid. It may be defined as that layer of fluid adjacent to a solid object in which the object surface has exerted its influence in the fluid through viscous drag. In the case of blood flow, it is the layer in which the fluid velocity increases as one moves away from the vessel wall (Figure 3.22).

Where there is parabolic laminar flow in a tube, the boundary layer extends all the way to the centre line of the tube. In the case of plug flow it is greatly reduced in thickness. And in the case of fully developed turbulent flow it is very thin, but will still exist as the fluid velocity is always zero at the wall itself.

Boundary layer separation

Boundary layer separation is the phenomenon of a boundary layer adjacent to an object over which the fluid flows becoming detached from that object to form a free boundary between two regions of flow (Figure 3.23). Boundary layer separation can occur at low or high Reynolds numbers. It will occur when the pressure gradient in the direction of flow increases and a region on the surface of the object develops a velocity moving in the opposite direction to the main flow. An increase in pressure may be expected where flow decelerates, for example, moving into a wider vessel.

In the case of a symmetrical obstacle and low Reynolds number flows (i.e. viscous forces predominate), boundary layer separation with an eddy will occur either side of the obstacle (Figure 3.23). This can occur for Reynolds numbers as low as 10. At high Reynolds number flows, reattachment of the boundary may not

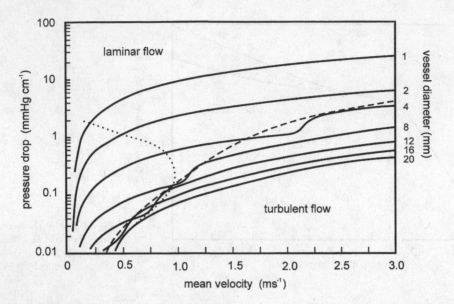

Figure 3.21 – Graph showing pressure drop against mean velocity for blood vessels of different diameters. Continuous flow is assumed. The line of critical velocities (Re = 2000) is marked (broken line) and an indication of normal peak systolic velocity for each vessel size is given (dotted line).

occur in a straightforward way. The eddy then propagates and develops oscillations, shedding vortices into the main flow, which can itself become fully turbulent. Generally speaking, regions of increasing pressure gradient and separated boundary layers also tend to be locations where disturbed flow can develop.

Flow through a stenosis

A stenosis is a narrowing of the arterial lumen, usually due to atheromatous plaque, that forms a resistance to

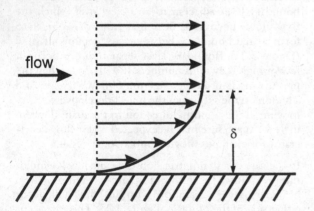

Figure 3.22 – Streamline diagram showing definition of boundary layer δ.

flow. Figure 3.24 shows a streamline diagram of flow through a stenosis and the Doppler waveforms seen at various locations. Qualitatively, the velocity of flow will increase as cross-sectional area A_1 decreases to A_2. Owing to the Bernoulli principle, the fluid pressure will drop at the entrance to the stenosis as potential energy is converted into kinetic energy. At the exit of the stenosis a fast jet extends into a wider vessel and so there will be a high Reynolds number and flow will be turbulent. In the case of pulsatile flow, turbulence will tend to form at peak systole when velocities are highest. It may propagate a considerable distance downstream. Distal to the stenosis at A_3 the pressure will tend to increase as the fluid velocity drops. Flow into a region of higher pressure is a condition that allows boundary layer separation with eddy formation to occur and this phenomenon is seen immediately distal to the stenosis. In stenoses where turbulence is produced, the change in vessel diameter at the exit may be increased by **post-stenotic dilatation**. This is believed to occur as a result of the turbulence causing vibrations in the vessel walls that alters their distensibility over time.

Next we look at the Doppler waveforms obtained around the stenosis using a long sample gate. Proximal to the stenosis the waveform is typical of the normal vessel with pulsatile flow and a parabolic-plug flow velocity profile. Within the stenosis the velocities are significantly higher than they were proximally, and the

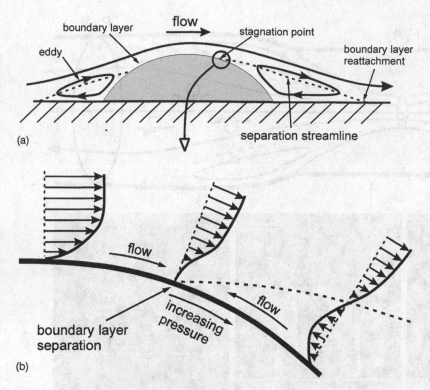

Figure 3.23 – Streamline diagram of continuous flow round a symmetrical obstacle (a) with a magnified view of the point of boundary layer separation (b).

velocity profile will be plug-turbulent depending on the actual flow conditions. Immediately distal to the stenosis there will be a fast jet that may be turbulent. This will show a high-velocity waveform with a ragged outline and complete filling of the systolic 'window'. Eddies will show up as bi-directional flow. This is because there actually is flow both towards and away from the ultrasound transducer within the sample volume. Turbulence will be heard on the audio signal.

Clinical note
Highest velocity

When examining flow through a stenosis it is important to note the highest velocity found, either in or immediately distal to the stenosis, as it is indicative of the degree of stenosis. Since the highest velocity may not be on the centre line of the vessel, it is good practice to use a sample volume long enough to include the whole lumen so that the highest velocity flow is not missed. In the case of asymmetric stenoses, the Doppler angle should be aligned with any jet seen rather than being aligned parallel to the vessel walls (Figure 3.25).

Turbulence in a stenosis

Figure 3.26 shows the critical velocity (Re = 2000) for different vessel diameters. In the case of **post-stenotic turbulence**, it is the vessel diameter distal to the stenosis that counts. Whether turbulence actually occurs will also depend on the surface contour of any plaque. Flow over a plaque with a smooth 'streamlined' contour is more likely to remain laminar than flow over an irregular ulcerated plaque that looks like the surface of the Moon.

Turbulence can be heard as an audible **bruit** through a stethoscope due to vibrations in the arterial wall caused by the disturbed flow.

Energy changes across a stenosis

Energy will be lost across a stenosis due to viscous loss as given by Poiseuille's equation and by inertial losses at the entrance and exit of the stenosis. The overall energy loss manifests itself as a pressure drop across the stenosis. The relative importance of these two components depends on the length of the stenoses and whether flow within the stenosis is laminar or turbulent. In mild degrees of stenoses the flow is more likely to be

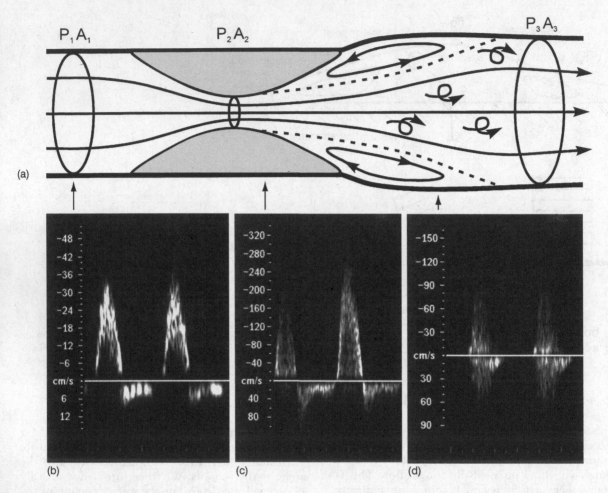

(a)

(b) (c) (d)

Figure 3.24 – Streamline diagram of flow through a stenosis with post stenotic dilatation of the vessel. Doppler spectra obtained at three points through the stenosis are shown.

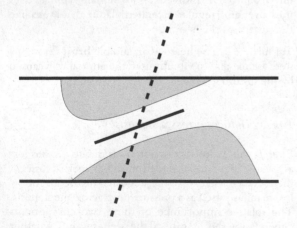

Figure 3.25 – Diagram showing correct positioning of angle cursor in an asymmetric stenosis.

laminar. This is also the case when there is generalised narrowing rather than a discrete stenosis. In these situations the pressure drop predicted by Poiseuille's equation will be the main loss. For discrete, relatively short high-grade stenoses, laminar flow will not exist either in or immediately distal to the stenosis and the losses will be almost entirely inertial losses. Because the velocity changes are likely to be large, these losses can be considerable.

Figure 3.27 shows the frictional loss as given by Poiseuille's equation for a 10-cm-long narrowing of a 6-mm diameter vessel. Figure 3.27a shows the pressure drop ΔP against the vessel radius for different volume flows. It shows the fourth power law for decreasing radius. Figure 3.27b shows the corresponding changes in velocity in the stenosis.

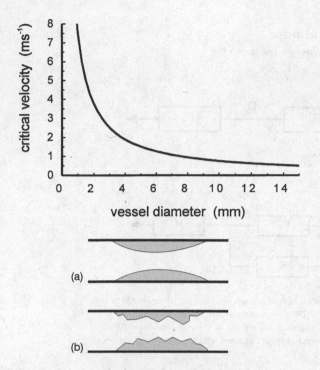

Figure 3.26 – Critical velocities (Re = 2000) for turbulence in a stenosis. The values of velocity indicated are likely to be lower when the stenosis has an uneven surface (b).

Figure 3.29 shows the pressure drop across a short stenosis caused by inertial loss. This loss arises principally because very little of the energy that is converted from pressure energy to increased velocity through the stenosis is recovered in the form of increased pressure distal to the stenosis (Bernoulli principle). It is lost as heat in turbulent flow. Since the losses arise from accelerating and decelerating the flow they are known as entrance and exit losses. They depend on the increase in kinetic energy in the stenosis and so the pressure drop is given by:

$$\Delta P = \frac{k\rho(v_s^2 - v_0^2)}{2} = \frac{k\rho Q}{2}\left(\frac{1}{a_s^2} - \frac{1}{a_0^2}\right)$$

where v_s is the velocity in the stenosis, v_0 is the velocity proximal to the stenosis, ρ is fluid density and k is a constant (≤ 1). Q is the volume flow and a_s, a_0 the respective cross-sectional areas. In Figure 3.28, k is set = 1 assuming no pressure is recovered distal to the stenosis. Note that from the volume flow equation $v^2 \propto 1/(\text{area})^2$, so that the inertial losses also depend on radius to the fourth power.

Figures 3.27 and 3.29 show the case where volume flow is kept constant through the stenosis. In an artery where there is a stenosis, the volume flow Q_0 to the peripheral vascular bed can only be kept constant if either the peripheral resistance R_p of the distal arterial tree is reduced to compensate for the increase in the resistance of the stenosis R_s, or there is a collateral route R_c (Figure 3.29b).

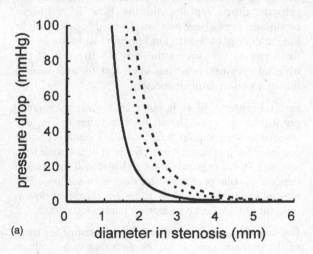

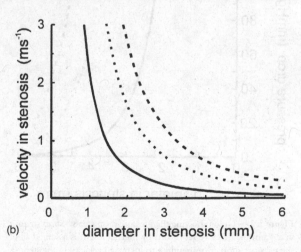

Figure 3.27 – Graphs showing a) viscous drop in pressure across a 10cm long narrowing in a 6mm diameter vessel. Each curve is for constant flow Q of 100 (solid line), 300 (dotted line) and 500 (broken line) ml min⁻¹, b) velocity in the stenosis corresponding to the same flows.

Technical note
Equations for flow through resistances

$$Q_0 = Q_s = \frac{\Delta P_{AV}}{R_{tot}}$$

$$R_{tot} = R_s + R_p$$

$$P_A - P_D = Q_0.R_s$$

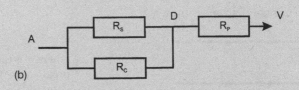

(a)

$$Q_0 = Q_s + Q_c = \frac{\Delta P_{AV}}{R_{tot}}$$

$$R_{tot} = \left(\frac{R_s R_c}{R_s + R_c}\right) + R_p$$

$$P_A - P_D = Q_0\left(\frac{R_s R_c}{R_s + R_c}\right)$$

$$Q_s = \frac{P_A - P_D}{R_s}$$

(b)

Figure 3.28 – Models of fluid resistances in an arterial supply (A) to a distal capillary bed (DV), a) when there is no collateral supply, and b) when there is a collateral supply. R_s is stenosis resistance, R_p is peripheral resistance and R_c is collateral resistance.

The overall changes in energy density across a stenosis are shown in Figure 3.30. This shows the energy changes for continuous flow through a model stenosis.

The top line of the shaded area is the total fluid energy at each point through the stenosis. As previously shown, most of the fluid energy in the proximal tube is in the form of fluid pressure with the kinetic energy of motion only accounting for a tiny fraction of the total. As the fluid moves into the stenosis it rapidly accelerates and pressure is converted into velocity. However, the sum of the pressure and kinetic energy drops and the fall in total energy is the entrance loss. Through the stenosis there is a pressure drop due to viscous losses described by Poiseuille's equation. At the exit, the velocity drops rapidly and the flow is turbulent producing a very large exit loss. The only conversion of kinetic energy back into fluid pressure is shown by the small rise in pressure at the exit. All the rest of the original pressure head has been lost to heat, sound (bruit) and non-laminar motion.

From Figure 3.30 it is clear that there is a large pressure drop across the stenosis and that in fact the viscous loss predicted by Poiseuille's equation only accounts for a relatively small fraction of the total loss. The size of the entrance and exit losses will very much depend on the geometry and degree of stenosis. The inertial losses are also likely to be greater when flow is pulsatile than when considering continuous flows.

Because the entrance and exit losses account for most of the pressure drop, it can be seen that two localised stenoses along a vessel are likely to be more significant than a single long one.

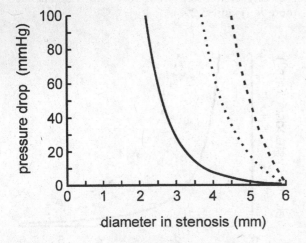

Figure 3.29 – Graph showing the pressure drop across a short stenosis in a 6mm diameter vessel caused by inertial loss. It is assumed all of the pressure drop corresponding to increased velocity in the stenosis is lost energy (k = 1). Each curve is for constant flow Q of 100 (solid line), 300 (dotted line) and 500 (broken line) ml min⁻¹.

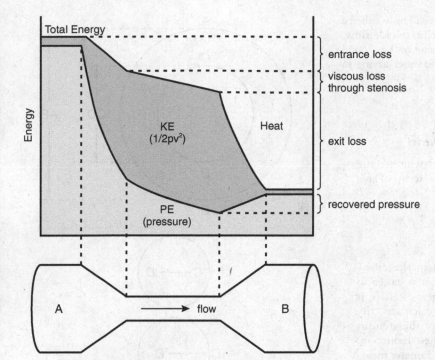

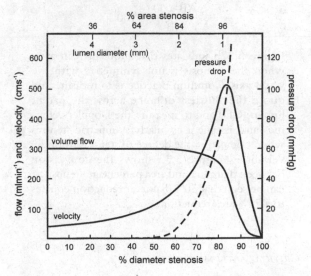

Figure 3.30 – Diagrammatic representation of energy losses occurring across a stenosis.

Significance of arterial stenosis

A stenosis caused by atheromatous plaque may be considered to be significant for two reasons: first, because of the effect it has on blood flow and, second, because of the presence of a plaque burden that may haemorrhage and embolise. The importance of this second factor will depend on the size and structure of the plaque and will not be discussed further here. Since the function of arteries is to carry oxygen to distal tissues, a stenosis can be described as significant if it reduces the volume flow, and hence the amount of oxygen being carried. A reduction in volume flow will also be accompanied by a reduction in distal perfusion pressure across the capillary bed.

Figure 3.31 illustrates what happens as a stenosis becomes tighter. At first the flow is maintained as the peak systolic velocity increases with little drop in pressure across the stenosis. As the degree of stenosis increases, flow becomes disturbed and the pressure drop begins to increase. At this point the volume flow then starts to decrease and flow to the distal capillary bed can only be maintained by vasodilation of the distal vessels. This change occurs when the vessel diameter is reduced by ~50%. At 50% stenosis the PSV has approximately doubled. (The velocity rises more slowly than the expected r^2 relationship with decreasing area because of the presence of turbulence.) For these reasons a 50%

diameter stenosis is usually considered to be haemodynamically significant and it can be detected by measuring a doubling of the peak velocity from that measured in the proximal vessel. At higher grades of stenosis the velocities continue to increase until at ~90–95% stenosis both the

Figure 3.31 – Graph showing volume flow, velocity and pressure drop at a stenosis in a 5mm diameter vessel. (based on data from Berger and Hwang (1973)[1], Spencer and Reid (1981)[8])

velocity and the flow become very small. This is called a **subocclusion** and the flow is described as **trickle flow**. The highest velocity reached will depend on how good the collateral flow is, i.e. is the stenotic vessel having to carry all the flow to the distal bed.

Clinical note
Percentage stenosis in arteries

It is important to be clear about whether the percentage stenosis is being given in terms of area or diameter reduction.

$$Q = A.\bar{v} = \frac{\pi D^2}{4}\bar{v}$$

Volume flow Q is proportional to the cross-sectional area A, but in practice it is easier to measure the diameter D of the vessel. It is therefore usual practice to calculate the percentage diameter reduction of the stenosis measured across the line of greatest reduction. This may then be compared with diameter measurements made from angiograms. Even when the degree of stenosis is being estimated using changes in velocity v, the values are still calculated for diameter reduction, rather than area, to give consistency and avoid confusion of results. The calculation is defined in Figure 3.32a:

$$\frac{AB-CD}{AB} \times 100$$

Figure 3.32b indicates that problems can arise when the stenosis is not symmetric with the vessel axis. Common practice is to measure and quote the shortest distance across the patent lumen (CD) and to measure the Doppler velocities and assume a circularly symmetric stenosis when calculating the degree of stenosis from the velocities. Figure 3.33 shows the conversion between diameter and area percentage stenosis. It can be seen that 50% diameter reduction equates to a 75% area reduction.

CRITICAL ARTERIAL STENOSIS

Another concept used is the idea of a **critical arterial stenosis**. This really refers to the clinical effect of the stenosis, with severe pain and tissue necrosis occurring

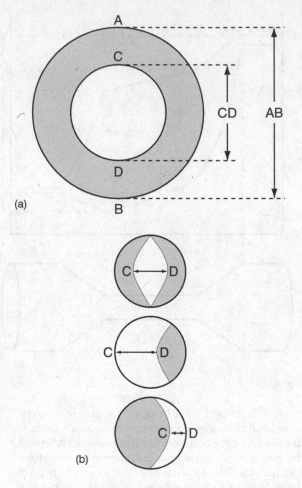

Figure 3.32 – a) Diagram defining distances to calculate percentage diameter reduction. b) Diagram illustrating the conventional way of measuring stenoses when disease is not symmetrical with the vessel axis.

due to **critical ischaemia**. A stenosis may be considered critical at rest when at ~80% diameter reduction very small increases in degree of stenosis cause a dramatic fall in blood flow. A stenosis that is not significant when the subject is at rest may become significant upon exercise when oxygen demand increases and blood flow tries to increase to supply the demand (Figures 3.27 and 3.28). Flow through the stenosis may then become more turbulent with a greater pressure drop due to entrance and exit losses. Clinically such a reduction in blood flow and oxygen supply produces pain known as **claudication** in the limbs and **angina** when referred to the heart. The pressure drop along an arterial segment may be measured at rest and after exercise to determine whether disease in the segment is significant at rest or only with higher flow following exercise.

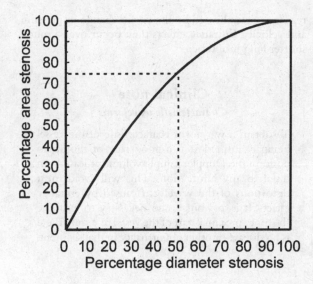

Figure 3.33 – Graph showing comparison of percentage area stenosis to percentage diameter stenosis.

Ankle brachial pressure index (ABPI) is calculated as the ratio of the arterial systolic pressure at ankle level to the brachial artery systolic pressure. It is used to give an indication of the severity of disease throughout the whole lower limb via the pressure drop caused by occlusive disease. By comparing the ankle pressure with the brachial pressure before and after exercise, the ankle pressure is normalised for any changes in systemic pressure there may be (Table 3.5).

STENOSED HEART VALVES

The drop in pressure across a stenosed heart valve may be estimated using the Bernoulli principle and calculating the drop in dynamic pressure P_D. The hydrostatic pressure terms cancel as there is no change in height. Velocity v_B is the highest velocity found in the stenotic jet, which is assumed to be in the valve itself and v_A is the velocity just proximal to the valve orifice:

$$P_{DA} - P_{DB} = \tfrac{1}{2}\rho \, (v_B^2 - v_A^2)$$

Table 3.5 – Ankle brachial pressure index

Normal	≥ 1
Mild disease	0.8–1.0
Moderate disease	0.6–0.8
Severe disease	0.4–0.6
Critical ischaemia	< 0.4

When expressed in millimetres of mercury, we have what is known as the **modified Bernoulli equation**:

$$\frac{1}{2} \cdot \frac{1060}{133.3} \, (v_B^2 - v_A^2) \qquad \text{i.e.} \qquad 4(v_B^2 - v_A^2) = \Delta P_D$$

As an estimate of pressure drop, it is based on the fact, shown above, that there is very little recovery of pressure distal to a stenosis. It also assumes that the stenosis is short enough and that there are no viscous losses as given by Poiseuille's equation. If $v_A \ll v_B$ this equation can be further simplified to (Table 3.6):

$$\Delta P_D = 4v_B^2$$

Entrance effects

What happens when the diameter of a vessel suddenly decreases at a particular location? Consider a large reservoir filled with fluid that is completely at rest with a tube coming out of the side (Figure 3.34). Fluid pressure in the reservoir will force fluid down the tube. We have already seen that steady flow in a tube will be laminar with a parabolic profile, so at some distance along the tube we may expect to see parabolic flow. However, at the entrance to the tube the velocity profile will be flat. This is because the pressure acts equally across the whole cross-sectional area and the stationary tube walls have not yet had any influence on the velocity profile. Figure 3.35 shows how the velocity profile will gradually become parabolic as the boundary layer adjacent to the tube wall extends further towards the centre line of the tube. This occurs as the stationary wall drags the fluid through viscous frictional forces, as previously discussed. The process of the boundary layer gradually growing away from the vessel wall is known as **viscous diffusion**. Near the entrance, the boundary layer grows in proportion to the square root of the distance from the entrance (x). The distance along the tube that it takes to become fully parabolic is known as

Table 3.6 – Typical guideline clinical values in aortic stenosis[4]

Degree of stenosis	Peak velocity (m s⁻¹)	Peak Doppler pressure drop (mmHg)	Valve area (cm²)†
Normal	1.4–2.2	8–20	> 3.0
Trivial	2.2–2.5	20–25	2.0–3.0
Mild	2.5–3.2	25–40	1.5–2.0
Moderate	3.2–4.2	40–70	1.0–1.5
Severe	> 4.2	> 70	< 1.0

†Calculated using the continuity equation.

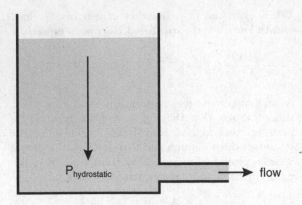

Figure 3.34 – Diagram of reservoir with an outlet pipe.

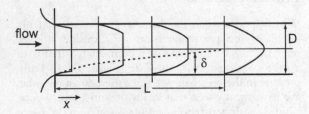

Figure 3.35 – Diagram showing velocity profiles and the development of a boundary layer (broken line) at the entrance to a tube.[2]

the entrance or **inlet length** L and depends on the vessel diameter D and Reynolds number (Re). For steady flow, L is approximately given by $0.003D$ Re and the thickness of the boundary layer:

$$\delta \propto \sqrt{\frac{xD}{\text{Re}}} = \sqrt{\frac{x\mu}{v\rho}}$$

Entrance effects are seen when there is a sudden decrease in vessel diameter, for example the branches of bifurcations and the proximal anastomoses of some grafts. They may also be seen when vessel walls begin to influence the flow of previously 'stationary' blood, for example the entrance to the aorta, and the systolic acceleration seen in some pulsatile waveforms.

- Aorta: $D = 0.026$ m, Re = ~3000, then $L = 2.3$ m

i.e. the whole of the aorta must be regarded as an entrance region.

- Superficial femoral artery (SFA): $D = 4$ mm, Re = 760, then $L = 0.14$ m

Note that these values are for steady laminar flow. In pulsatile flow the behaviour of flow in an entrance region is complicated by the cyclic change in pressure and velocity. Entrance effects then occur over a much shorter length of tube.

Fluid jets

We now consider the opposite case, of flow from a small orifice into a reservoir of fluid at rest. The result is a fluid jet that will show turbulence even at very low Reynolds numbers (Figure 3.36). Typically, Re > 10 will produce turbulent flow in this situation. Near to the orifice the flow will depend on the geometry of the orifice and the jet retains the cross-sectional shape of the orifice. This feature enables an estimate of the orifice size to be made by measuring the width of the base of the jet as shown by colour-flow imaging. There is a free boundary layer between the fluid in the jet and the surrounding static fluid. In this situation the shear flow along the boundary layer quickly becomes unstable and eddies form. Very small eddies along the boundary layer will transfer their energy into the adjacent stationary fluid by viscous frictional forces. By this means the jet spreads out in a cone shape away from the orifice, a process called **entrainment**. Although the jet spreads out linearly, the actual boundary is very irregular along this line. Small eddies are formed around the edges of larger eddies. These larger eddies have higher velocities and are governed by inertial forces rather than by viscous forces. They carry the main energy within the jet forward for a considerable distance away from the orifice. The length of the jet as shown by colour-flow imaging therefore gives a second indication of the significance of the flow through an orifice. The energy in the jet is dissipated relatively slowly by an energy cascade from the larger eddies through to the small then tiny eddies where viscous losses predominate. These processes are also responsible for the propagation of turbulence downstream from a stenosis when Re is high. Fluid jets are

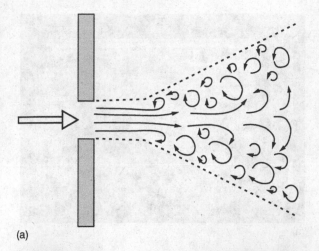

(a)

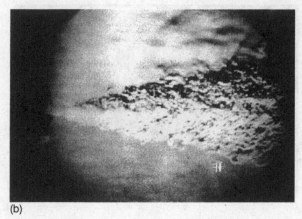

(b)

Figure 3.36 – a) Streamline diagram of flow in a turbulent jet. b) Schlieren picture of a two-dimensional jet in water, obtained by having the jet at a slightly different temperature from ambient.[11]

seen in the right ventricle in the presence of septal defects, distal to very tight stenoses and adjacent to regurgitant valves.

Flow in curved tubes

When fluid flows through a curved tube, centrifugal force F_c acting on the mass of fluid must be considered in addition to the inertial and viscous forces considered so far. This is the force that pushes someone in a car to the outside of the bend when taking a corner quickly. It depends on the mass, or density ρ, for a fluid, the velocity v and radius of curvature r_c of the tube:

$$F_c = \frac{\rho v^2}{r}$$

Centrifugal force will therefore be greatest on the fluid with the greatest velocity, which for a straight tube is the stream along the centre line of the tube. Along this axis centrifugal force dominates the pressure forces within the fluid, forcing the fluid toward the outer edge of the bend. Near the tube wall viscous forces slow the fluid and pressure forces predominate and induce a circumferential motion round the walls towards the inside of the bend. This combination of forces sets up two helical vortices spaced symmetrically about the plane of curvature of the tube (Figure 3.37).

These helical vortices will influence the distribution of axial velocity so that the maximum velocity will move away from the centre line of the tube toward the outer edge of the bend (Figure 3.38).

This type of flow is seen in the aortic arch (Figure 3.38b), at bifurcations, where the axial streamlines must move outwards from the vessel centre into the branches, and in tortuous vessels.

Clinical note
Kinks and coils in carotid arteries

Figure 3.39 shows a tortuous internal carotid artery with a sharp kink. The peak systolic velocity at the outside of the bend (c) is higher than that at the inside of the bend (b). Sharp kinks such as this have been associated with cerebral transient ischaemic events even in the absence of atheromatous disease. This may be associated with the high shear rates adjacent to the vessel walls that occur in such bends. Such tortuosity is more commonly found in older subjects. By comparison, coiling in the manner of a corkscrew sometimes seen in young as well as old subjects is probably congenital and appears to be benign.

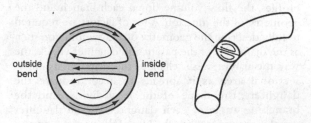

outside bend   inside bend

Figure 3.37 – Diagram showing the secondary flows that develop as fluid flows along a curved tube.[7]

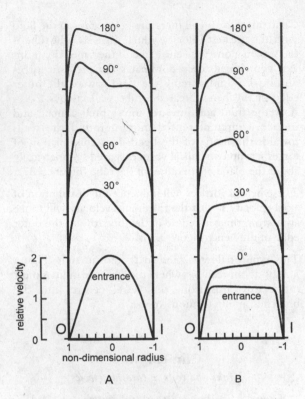

Figure 3.38 – Diagram showing the velocity profiles that develop as fluid flows along a curved tube a) where the profile at entry is parabolic and b) where there is a blunt entrance profile as would be seen in the aorta. The angle round the bend is indicated.[7]

Bifurcations

In the course of supplying all the peripheral tissues, the arteries divide many times. In the majority of junctions the parent artery splits into two daughter vessels forming a bifurcation. With the exception of the aortic bifurcation, which splits symmetrically into the iliac arteries and the pulmonary artery, most bifurcations are asymmetric. The flow patterns seen in bifurcations are complex and depend on the proximal velocity profiles, the flow volume down each branch and the geometry of the junction. A lot of factors are required to fully describe the geometry of a given junction such as the diameters of the parent and daughter vessels, the way the parent vessel changes the shape of its cross-sectional area as it spreads to accommodate the daughters, the shape of the flow divider and the branching angle of each daughter. As the daughter vessel moves away from the line of the parent, a curved segment of vessel is formed and we may expect to see the sort of flow patterns described for flow in curved

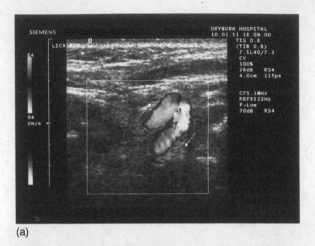

(a)

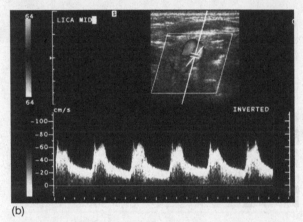

(b)

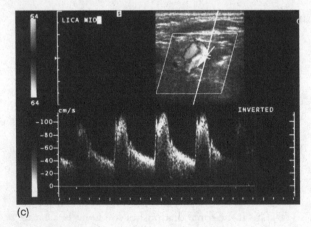

(c)

Figure 3.39 – Images and Doppler waveforms seen in a tortuous internal carotid artery. a) Direction of flow round a sharp kink. b) Waveform from inside bend. c) Waveform from outside bend.

tubes. Figure 3.40 shows qualitatively the flow patterns seen in a symmetrical bifurcation for laminar flow conditions (Re = 100–1400) and the same peripheral resistance in each branch.

The velocity profiles are shown in the upper branch and the boundary flows and secondary motions in the lower branch for clarity. The actual flow in both branches will be the same.

The features seen all result from the flow phenomena already discussed. At the point where the flow meets the flow divider, fast axial streamlines will immediately be adjacent to a vessel wall. A new boundary layer must develop along this wall as in entrance-type flow conditions. The shear stress adjacent to the wall will be high as the boundary layer builds up through viscous forces. On the opposite wall, the streamlines will have to turn round the bend and may become detached from the wall to form a separation zone with a free boundary layer. This then gives a region of low shear stress where velocities are low and change slowly. Because the daughter branch moves away from the line of the parent axis, there is effectively a curved segment of vessel and secondary motions will develop as a result of centrifugal force. As in curved tubes, the secondary helical vortices move the point of fastest flow towards the outside of the bend. This explains the solid velocity profile seen in the upper branch. In the plane perpendicular to the plane of the bifurcation the velocity profile will have a dip along the vessel axis.

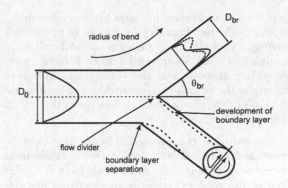

Figure 3.40 – Diagram showing the velocity profiles, secondary flows and boundary layers that are seen around a symmetrical bifurcation. Velocity profiles are shown in upper branch, solid line in plane of bifurcation, broken line in orthogonal plane.[7]

The two velocity profiles are more clearly appreciated when seen in relation to a contour map of the velocity across the daughter vessel lumen (Figure 3.41). Each contour is a line of constant velocity.

Asymmetric bifurcations are more common in the arterial system. Their asymmetry may arise from:

- different cross-sectional area;
- different branching angle; or
- different flows in each of the branches.

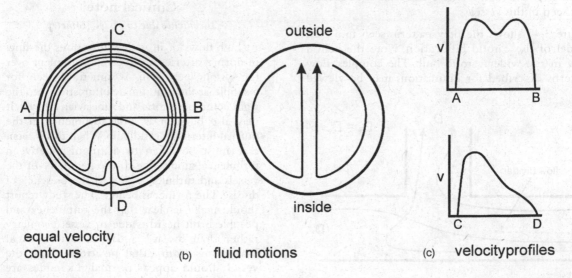

(a) equal velocity contours   (b) fluid motions   (c) velocity profiles

Figure 3.41 – Diagrams showing a) equal velocity contours, b) fluid motions and c) velocity profiles occurring in each branch of a symmetrical bifurcation.[7]

In general, flow separation is most likely to occur in the smaller of the two branches. In the case of one branch having zero branching angle, there will still be a complex three-dimensional flow pattern with secondary motions near the walls. Streamlines may move past the branch exit before doubling back round the walls of the parent vessel to flow down the branch (Figure 3.42).

In this situation two separation zones may form. S_1 results as flow negotiates a sharp corner. S_2 results from the sideways flow into the side branch. Flow along this wall of the tube experiences an increasing pressure gradient distal to the branching point and flow separation will occur. Boundary layer reattachment to the wall usually occurs within 2.5 vessel diameters of the junction, and in pulsatile flow the separation zone usually only exists over part of the cycle.

The existence of low shear separation zones, where blood is less mobile, and regions of higher shear where endothelial erosion can occur accounts for the fact that bifurcations are frequently the sites where atheromatous disease is found. In measurements made on dogs, endothelial damage has been seen when shear stresses > 37.9 Pa exist. In normal flows, shear stresses in the aorta of 4–27 Pa were seen, and up to 36 Pa was seen in the coronary arteries. These values are not far short of those necessary to cause damage. Higher values may be found near the flow divider of bifurcations. Low shear rates seen on the outer wall of the carotid bulb occur over the region where atheroma is frequently first seen in this vessel.

Figure 3.43 shows the flow patterns seen in a glass model of the carotid bifurcation. Note the helical flow in the wider carotid bulb. The complex flow patterns described for bifurcations may be viewed

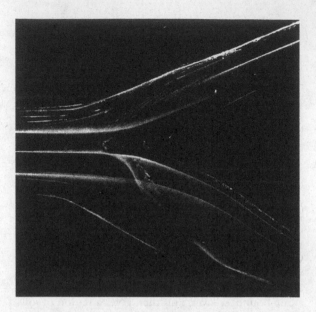

Figure 3.43 – Photo of streamlines a glass tube model of the carotid bifurcation showing the complex secondary motions occurring in the carotid bulb.[12]

using colour Doppler cineloop. The changes in flow pattern may be examined frame by fame across the cardiac cycle.

Clinical note
Turbulence due to vessel geometry

At high flows or in wide bifurcations the flow in normal arteries may become turbulent over the systolic peak. This is sometimes seen, for example, at the innominate bifurcation into the right common carotid and subclavian arteries. It may also be seen as spike turbulence in the normal internal carotid bulb. When this is seen, care must be taken to distinguish between turbulence simply due to the geometry of the vessels and turbulence due to the presence of disease. The former is benign. The study report should make it clear that the turbulence and possible bruit heard is due to vessel geometry rather than disease, and that it is normal. Waveforms from distal positions along the vessel should appear normal. Examples are shown in Figure 3.44.

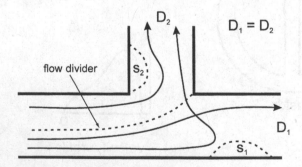

Figure 3.42 – Diagram showing streamlines and separation zones occurring at a right angled bifurcation.[7]

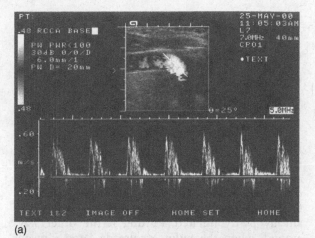

(a)

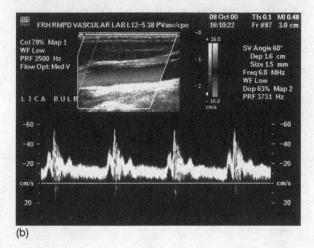

(b)

Figure 3.44 – Doppler waveforms showing turbulence due to geometry. a) Proximal common carotid artery with normal calibre lumen. b) Normal internal carotid bulb.

Clinical note
Position of a sample volume

Because of the complex flow patterns seen in bifurcations, strongly curved vessels and aneurysmal vessels, unusual or atypical waveforms may be obtained from them. Usually a slight repositioning of the sample volume within the vessel lumen will produce a more normal looking waveform. The use of a longer sample volume may also help as the fastest flow is often shifted away from the vessel centre line.

Confluence of veins

Apart from the presence of valves, the other distinguishing feature of veins is that flow at bifurcations runs in the opposite sense to that seen in most arteries. There is a confluence of flow from the branches into a larger parent vessel (Figure 3.45). At the junction, slow flow adjacent to the wall moves into the centre stream of the parent vessel. This causes two pairs of secondary vortices to form as the fast centre-stream as flow from each branch is forced to turn into the parent vessel and may be seen at the junction of the inferior vena cava with the common iliac veins.

Vessel diameters

The walls of real arteries are elastic. The radius of the vessel will therefore increase with higher blood pressure in the same way as the inner tube of a bicycle tyre does when inflated. The blood pressure within the vessel P_i is balanced by the **extramural pressure** outside the vessel P_o and the **tension** T developed within the vessel wall. Tension is the force per unit length acting along the line of circumference round the vessel. The difference between the blood pressure and the extramural pressure is known as the **transmural pressure** P_{tm}. The absolute tension in the wall depends on the wall elasticity and any muscle tone developed within the wall. It must be found from measurements of real vessels. This will then determine the vessel radius r for a given transmural pressure (Figure 3.46a). The relationship between these quantities is called Laplace's law:

$$T = P_{tm}r \ (\text{N m}^{-1})$$

Laplace's Law

which is useful for considering relative changes from measured values.

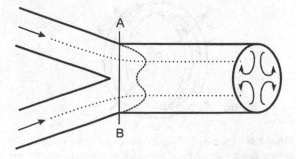

Figure 3.45 – Diagram showing the secondary motions set up at the confluence of two veins. The velocity profile across AB is also shown.

In the body at rest, the extramural pressure is usually close to atmospheric pressure and can be taken as zero. However, the external pressure may be positive, tending to compress the vessel, for example a vessel in a contracting muscle where the extramural pressure may be greater than systolic pressure. Or it may be negative and below atmospheric pressure, enhancing the effects of the internal fluid pressure, for example vessels in the thoracic cavity during inhalation. During respiration the pressure in the thorax varies by ±23 mmHg about atmospheric pressure.

If we look at a vessel with wall thickness h, we need to consider the circumferential force per unit area exerted by the vessel wall called the **circumferential stress** S_w (Figure 3.46b):

$$S_w = \frac{P_{tm} r}{h} \ (Nm^{-2} = Pa)$$

Circumferential Stress

The wall thickness h changes in such a way that the cross-sectional area of the wall when viewed in transverse section remains constant. In the smaller arteries and arterioles the circumferential stress may be actively increased above that due to the basic wall elasticity by

the activation of smooth muscle in the wall. The radius of the vessel will therefore change:

- if the transmural pressure changes; or

- if the stress in the vessel wall changes through the active contraction of smooth muscle or through structural changes in the elastic components of the vessel wall.

Laplace's law shows that the increase in pressure required to increase the radius by a fixed amount against a given wall tension is greater for a small radius than a large radius ($T/\Delta r = \Delta P$). This is why it is harder to blow up a balloon when it is small than when it is already partly inflated. Putting it the other way around, when the radius is already large a given increase in pressure will increase the radius much further than when the vessel was small. A much larger increase in wall tension is then required to balance the increase in pressure and radius. Eventually the tension will exceed the elastic integrity of the wall and it will rupture. This can be prevented if the wall tension increases more rapidly, as the vessel radius increases, than simple elastic theory predicts. It is equivalent to saying that the wall must become less compliant and more rigid as the radius increases. This is exactly what happens in real vessels where the walls have both elastic elastin fibres and stiffer collagen fibres withstanding stress in the wall. The effect of the elastin and collagen fibres within the vessel wall combine to produce a non-linear radius versus pressure curve (Figure 3.47).

At low pressures the vessel wall stress is supported by the elastic behaviour of elastin and the curve is linear. At high pressures the wall stress is supported by the more rigid collagen fibres and the increase in radius is limited. This arrangement has been likened to an elastic balloon inside a string bag that limits the expansion of the balloon.

The increase in radius over the original radius $\Delta r/r$ is known as **strain**. The related curve (Figure 3.48a) is therefore known as a **stress–strain curve**.

Figure 3.48 also shows the effect of increasing smooth muscle tone in the vessel wall. The wall becomes stiffer so the stress for a given radius is increased (Figure 3.48a) and at any given pressure the radius is reduced (Figure 3.48b). It is by increasing smooth muscle tone that the radius of smaller arteries, and hence peripheral resistance to flow, may be controlled by the sympathetic nervous system.

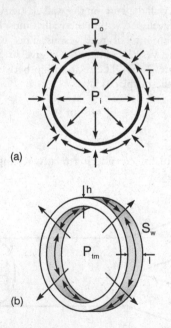

(a)

(b)

Figure 3.46 – Diagram defining a) Laplace's law where T is vessel wall tension, P_i is intramural blood pressure, P_o is extramural pressure and b) tangential stress S_w for transmural pressure P_{tm}, wall thickness h and vessel elemental length l.

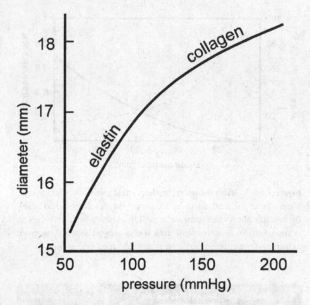

Figure 3.47 – Change in diameter of human abdominal aorta with increasing pressure.[5]

The change in vessel diameter with change in blood pressure over the cardiac cycle can be viewed using an M-mode ultrasound display. An example taken from a normal internal carotid bulb is shown in Figure 3.49. (Further data are given in Appendix D.)

Aneurysm

In the case of an aneurysm, the structural integrity of the vessel wall is compromised and the radius increases significantly. This is the equivalent of a weak point in a bicycle inner-tube bulging out. Figure 3.50 shows the theoretical circumferential wall stresses in an abdominal aortic aneurysm. The blood pressure is constant at 150 mmHg. Note that as the vessel diameter increases from 1.4 to 10 cm (×7.3), the wall stress increases by a factor of 57. Someone with a 10 cm aortic aneurysm has a 60% chance of rupture being the cause of death.[12] A large aneurysm is very pulsatile as the change in radius over the change in pressure, from systolic to diastolic, is also large.

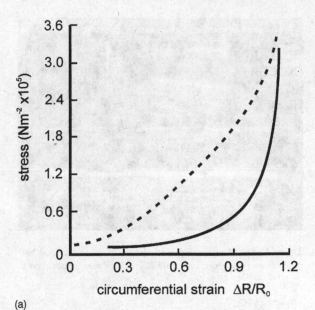

(a)

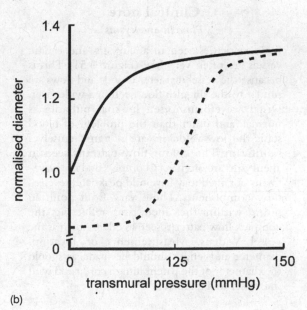

(b)

Figure 3.48 – Graphs showing a) stress-strain curve for canine carotid artery in-vitro (R_0 is activated radius at P_{tm} = 25mmHg), b) change in normalised diameter (relative to diameter at zero pressure with no smooth muscle activation) as transmural pressure is increased in canine iliac artery in-vitro. Solid curves show changes with smooth muscle inactivated. Broken lines show changes after stimulation of smooth muscle with noradrenaline.[3]

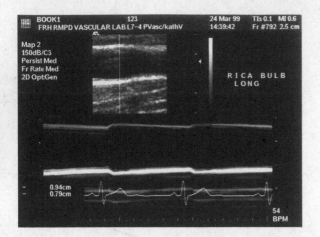

Figure 3.49 – M-mode display of change in internal carotid bulb diameter over the cardiac cycle. An ECG trace is shown for comparison.

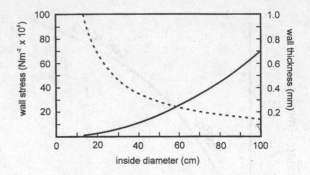

Figure 3.50 – Graph showing the theoretical values for wall stress in a human abdominal aorta as an aneurysm develops (solid line). Broken line shows the decrease in wall thickness which decreases so as to maintain constant wall area when viewed in cross-section. Transmural pressure remains constant at 150 mmHg.

Clinical note
Flow in aneurysms

Flow velocities seen in aneurysms and ectatic vessels are often very low (Figure 3.51). This is because the vessel diameter is wide and flows are similar to the sluggish flow seen in a wide river. Distal waveforms often look as pulsatile as normal, and other than the problem of blood stasis the low velocities are not in themselves significant. The colour-flow patterns seen in aneurysms are often very complex and the waveforms obtained may have odd peaks and reverse-flow components. These vary from point to point within the aneurysm, reflecting the complex flow patterns seen as eddies form as the vessel widens. Measurements of location, diameter and length should be made, as should the diameter of the patent lumen compared with the vessel wall diameter.

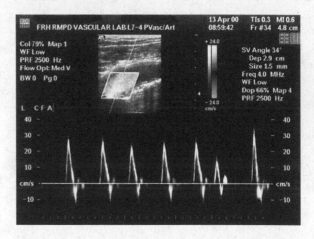

Figure 3.51 – Doppler waveforms obtained from an ectatic common femoral artery. PSV is only 30 cms^{-1} compared with a normal value of >50 cms^{-1}, but waveform shape is normal.

Heart wall

In the case of the muscular walls of heart chambers, it is the stress developed in the walls as the muscle tone is increased that raises the blood pressure within each chamber. This is the mechanism by which the heart puts energy into the blood to drive it round the circulation. Laplace's law applies to the heart, but the circumferential wall stress must now be considered in two orthogonal directions (Figure 3.52). Full analysis of the forces is complicated by the thickness of the heart wall, the complex volume shape of the ventricles and the structural arrangement of the muscle fibres.

Vessel collapse

A large increase in extramural pressure, an increase in wall stress by smooth muscle tone or a drop in internal fluid pressure will lead to a vessel collapsing so all flow ceases. In the case of a decrease in transmural pressure, once the vessel elasticity is completely relaxed further decrease in pressure will cause the vessel cross-section

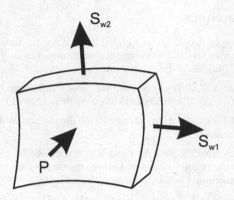

Figure 3.52 – Diagram showing two orthogonal wall stresses that occur as pressure develops in the ventricles of the heart.

to change from circular to elliptical, and then to collapse to form two small parallel channels. Complete occlusion may occur as irregularities of the vessel wall seal off the residual lumen (Figure 3.53).

Venous pressures

The transmural pressure range over which veins collapse is ±7.5 mmHg (-10^3 to $+10^3$ N m^{-2}) (Figure 3.53). This is in the middle of the physiological range. The cross-sectional area of veins therefore varies considerably with pressure changes due to respiration, hydrostatic changes with changes in posture, changes in skeletal muscle tone and arteriolar smooth muscle tone. These are important factors in changing the total volume of the venous space in the circulation and give it an important function as the volume reservoir of the circulation.

Starling resistor

There are a number of sites in the body where flow through the capillary bed is modulated by changes in the extramural pressure. This arrangement, of an extramural pressure regulating the resistance of a thin-walled collapsible vessel, has been used experimentally and is known as a **Starling resistor** (Figure 3.54). Examples of blood flow being regulated in this manner are in the liver during respiration and intracerebral flow following trauma.

Systolic pressure measurement

The principle of applying a high extramural pressure to collapse a vessel is used to measure blood pressure with a sphygmomanometer. The cuff is inflated to a pressure greater than systolic pressure, thereby occluding the artery. Pressure in the cuff is measured, for example, by a column of mercury (Figure 3.6). As the cuff is deflated, the pressure where flow recommences is detected by a hand-held Doppler probe, or the sound of the turbulent jet is listened for with a stethoscope. This determines the peak systolic pressure in the vessel, which is the fluid pressure just able to open the artery against the extramural cuff pressure, and flow commences down the artery.

Mechanics of valves

The proper functioning of both the aortic and venous valves depends on the shape of the vessel at the valve and the flow patterns that develop around it (Figure 3.55). Immediately behind the attachment point of

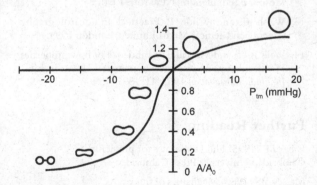

Figure 3.53 – Graph showing the change in cross-sectional area of a vein as transmural pressure varies over the physiological range. The area is shown relative to the area A_0 at zero transmural pressure.[4]

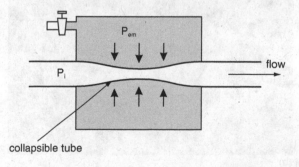

Figure 3.54 – Diagram of a Starling resistor. The resistance to flow in the collapsible tube is controlled by running fluid into or out of the extramural compartment thereby varying the extramural pressure P_{em}.

the valve leaflets is a widening of the vessel to form a **sinus**. In the case of the aortic valve these are known as the sinuses of Valsalva. As forward flow through the valve commences, the valve leaflets are pushed back towards the vessel wall and an eddy develops behind the leaflet within the sinus. The leaflets are held in the open position by a balance of pressure of the forward flow on one side and the sinus eddy on the other. When flow reverses, flow moving into the sinus behind the leaflet swiftly pushes the leaflets together, closing the valve. If the sinuses were not present and the leaflets were pushed flush against the vessel wall by forward flow, the efficiency of valve closure would be greatly reduced with reflux occurring before valve closure. As it is, the valve is very sensitive to back pressure and virtually no reflux occurs before valve closure. During forward flow the leaflets follow the line of the vessel wall so there is no obstruction to flow by the leaflets. The valves of the heart are discussed in more detail in Chapter 5.

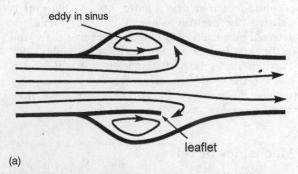

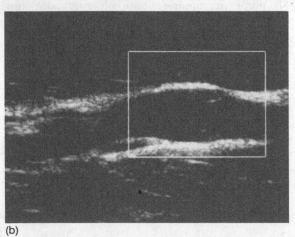

Figure 3.55 – a) Streamline diagram of flow through a valve with the valve leaflets in the open position. b) Image of an upper limb vein valve with flow from right to left.

References

1. Berger R and Hwang NHC. Critical arterial stenosis: a theoretical and experimental solution. *Annals of Surg* 1974; **180**: 39–50.

2. Caro CG, Pedley TJ, Schroter RC, Seed WA. The mechanics of the circulation. Oxford University Press, Oxford 1978.

3. Milnor WR. Hemodynamics. Williams and Wilkins, Baltimore 1982.

4. Moreno AH, Katz AI, Gold RD, Reddy RV. Mechanics of distension of veins and other very thin walled tubular structures. *Circulation Research* 1970; **27**: 1069–1080.

5. Nichols WW and O'Rourke MF. McDonald's blood flow in arteries (4th edition). Arnold, London 1998.

6. Oates CP, Williams ED, McHugh MI. The use of a Diasonics DRF400 duplex ultrasound scanner to measure volume flow in arterio-venous fistulae in patients undergoing haemodialysis: an assessment of measurement uncertainties. *Ultrasound in Med. & Bioil.* 1990; **16**: 571–579.

7. Pedley TJ. The fluid mechanics of large blood vessels. Cambridge University Press, Cambridge 1980.

8. Spencer MP and Reid JM (eds). Cerebrovascular evaluation with ultrasound. Martinus Nijhoff, The Hague 1981.

9. Stonebridge PA and Ruckley CV. Abdominal aortic aneurysms: in *A textbook of vascular medicine*, Tooke JE and Lowe GDO (eds) Arnold, London 1996.

10. Summer DS. The hemodynamics and pathophsiology of arterial disease: in *Vascular Surgery*, Rutherford RB (ed) WB Saunders 1977.

11. Tritton DJ. Physics fluid dynamics Oxford University Press, Oxford 1988.

12. Van Steenhoven AA, Rindt CCM, Reneman RS, Janssen JD. Numerical and experimental analysis of carotid artery blood flow: in *Biomechanical Transport Processes*, Mosora F (ed) plenum, New York 1990.

13. Walsh C and Wilde P. Practical Echocardiography Greenwich Medical Media Limited, London 1999.

14. Wells RTE and Merrill EW. Influence of flow properties of blood upon viscosity-hematocrit relationships. *J Clinical Investigation* 1962; **41**: 1591–1598.

Further Reading

Faber TE (1995) Fluid dynamics for physicists Cambridge University Press, Cambridge

Massey BS (1983) Mechanics of fluids Van Nostrand Reinhold (UK) Co. Ltd, Wokingham

Tritton DJ (1988) Physics fluid dynamics Oxford University Press, Oxford

4

PULSATILE FLOW

PULSATILE FLOW

Outline

The complex pulse pressure and flow waves seen in real arteries are shown to consist of the sum of simple harmonic waves. Their behaviour in vessels is described with reference to the Wormersley parameter α. Features associated with the propagation of waves are examined including wave energy, vascular impedance and reflections, and their effects on Doppler waveforms is indicated. Velocity profiles, turbulent flow and damped waveforms are discussed. Flow in veins is described.

So far we have only considered those aspects of flow that describe continuous flow in a rigid tube. This has enabled us to understand many of the effects of a change in vessel diameter, where the flow seen is governed by the Bernoulli principle, Poiseuille's equation and Reynolds number. We now turn our attention to consider pulsatile flow in tubes with elastic walls such as are found in real arteries. First, we look at how the shape of the waveform envelope arises, then, second, at the velocity profiles seen in pulsatile flow. That will explain the distribution of grey levels seen in arterial waveforms. Finally the waveforms in veins will be looked at.

Pulse pressure and flow wave

Blood is an incompressible fluid, so as the left ventricle of the heart contracts and the aortic valve opens, blood in the ascending aorta experiences a rapid rise in pressure as the stroke volume of the left ventricle is pushed into the aorta. This is followed by a fall in pressure in the left ventricle until the aortic valve closes when the aortic pressure exceeds that of the ventricle. The rapid rise in pressure causes the elastic vessel wall of the aorta to bulge out locally with an increase in radius of 6–8%, as described by Laplace's equation. It then rebounds as the pressure falls and the overall effect is to produce a pressure pulse that moves off along the aorta and into the whole arterial circulation (Figure 4.1).

The relative motion of the vessel wall is analogous to having two ropes laid out in parallel on a flat surface

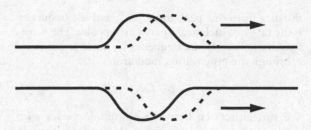

Figure 4.1 – Principle of a pulse pressure wave travelling along an artery.

and then giving them a sudden shake in opposite directions. A wave of increased spacing will be seen to travel away down the ropes. In arteries this is called the **pulse pressure wave**.

Pulse flow wave and the velocity waveform

Accompanying the pulse pressure wave will be a **pulse flow wave** as the blood moves in response to the changes in pressure. It is the velocity $v(t)$ of this pulse flow wave $Q(t)$, as given by the volume flow equation, that is the familiar **Doppler velocity waveform** displayed by an ultrasound scanner:

$$Q(t) = A.v(t)$$

where A is the vessel cross-sectional area.

Note: the **flow waveform** will have the same shape as the **velocity waveform** as seen on the Doppler spectral display. The only difference between them is that the unit of velocity is m s⁻¹ and the unit of volume flow is m³ s⁻¹. Numerically the difference is the scaling factor of the cross-sectional area as given by the volume flow equation. If this is remembered, confusion between the two terms can be avoided.

Basic waveform theory

If we take, for example, the pressure variation in a pure tone sound wave travelling through air or a simple oscillating pulse pressure wave travelling along an artery and draw a graph of pressure variation, we produce the familiar picture of a sine wave (Figure 4.2). The wave shape is also known as **simple harmonic motion**. Such a simple harmonic travelling wave is fully described by its **frequency** f, **amplitude** a_0 and **wavelength** λ. The amplitude is the size of the disturbance, the wavelength is the distance from one peak to the next and the frequency is the rate at which peaks pass a given point. The wavelength is related to the frequency by the speed of travel c through the propagating medium:

$$c = f.\lambda$$

We can either see how the amplitude varies with distance through the medium (Figure 4.2a) or can observe at one point and watch how the amplitude varies with time (Figure 4.2b).

Notice that after one wavelength has passed, the variation of the amplitude repeats itself. This is like going round a circle, when after one circuit the journey repeats itself. One wavelength is therefore also known as one cycle and the distance can be measured along it in degrees from 0 to 360 as for distance round a circle. The sine (sin (ϕ)) of angle ϕ at each point then gives the amplitude of the wave at that point, hence the name 'sine wave'. Instead of degrees we could use radians where 360° is 2π radians and 90° is $\pi/2$ radians. The angular distance along a wave is known as its **phase** ϕ, and the rate or frequency at which 2π radians is completed is known as the **angular frequency**

$$\omega = 2\pi f$$

The timing of two waveforms may be compared with one another by means of their frequency and phase ϕ.

For example, Figure 4.3a and b shows two similar sine waves whose frequency is the same, but whose phase differs by 90°. Here the phase of (b) leads (is ahead of) (a) by 90°. Now, this is a particularly important case to note. With a phase lead of 90° the wave in (b) describes the **gradient** or slope of the wave in (a). It has its maximum amplitude when the slope of (a) is steepest and is zero when (a) changes from a positive to a negative going slope. It exactly maps out the changing slope of (a). It will be shown below that in an ideal situation, this is the phase relationship between the pulse flow wave and the pulse pressure wave. Figure 4.3c shows a sine wave of lower frequency but whose phase at the start of the observation t_0, is the same as that for (a).

The amplitude a, angular frequency ω and phase ϕ of a simple sine wave are related through the sine wave equation:

$$a = a_0 \sin (\omega t - \phi)$$

Sine Wave Equation

where a is calculated with reference to the waveform $a_0 \sin (\omega t)$ (Figure 4.4) shown as the broken line that

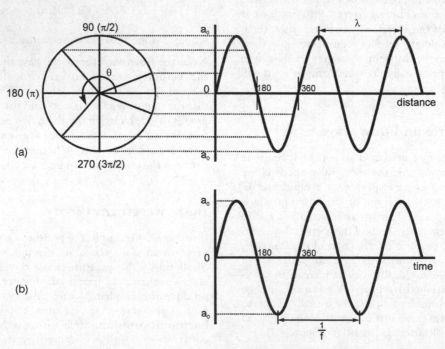

Figure 4.2 – Travelling sine wave as (a) variation of amplitude with distance and (b) variation of amplitude with time. The relationship between one cycle of a sine wave and travelling once round a circular path is also shown.

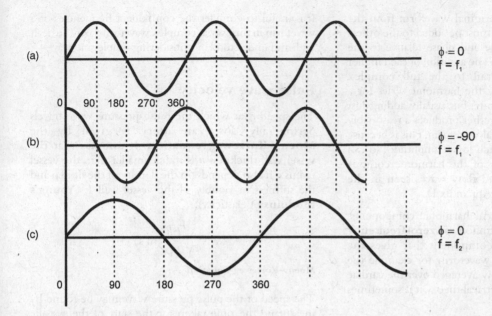

(a) $\phi = 0$
$f = f_1$

(b) $\phi = -90$
$f = f_1$

(c) $\phi = 0$
$f = f_2$

Figure 4.3 – Three sine waves with different phases ϕ: (a, b) have the same frequency f_1, but their phase differs by 90°; (a, c) have different frequencies f_1, f_2, but their initial phases are the same.

'begins' its cycle at $t = 0$. The phase angle $\phi = \omega t_0$, where t_0 is the difference in time between the waveform we wish to calculate and the reference waveform. If the phase is negative the waveform **lags** (is later than) the reference waveform (Figure 4.4a). If the phase is positive (Figure 4.4b) the waveform **leads** (is ahead of) the reference waveform.

Component frequencies of a complex waveform

Looking at the more complex waveforms seen in real arteries, it is known that the whole waveform shape repeats itself every cardiac cycle. This is true for both the pulse pressure wave and the flow wave. The basic or **fundamental frequency** of these complex waveforms is therefore equal to the heart rate. However, these waveforms do have a more complex shape than a simple sine wave that repeats itself every cardiac cycle. Fourier's theory shows that any repeating complex waveform, such as we see in the pulse pressure wave or a Doppler velocity waveform, may be constructed by adding together simple sine waves of different frequencies and phases. In particular, it allows the complex waveform to be analysed and described by a series of simple component sine waves known as **harmonics**. The lowest frequency of such a series is known as the **fundamental** or first harmonic. It has the same frequency as the repetition frequency of the complex waveform, which for arterial waveforms is the heart rate. The second and third harmonics will be at two times and three times the frequency of the first harmonic, and so on for higher harmonics. Fourier analysis determines the amplitude and phase of each

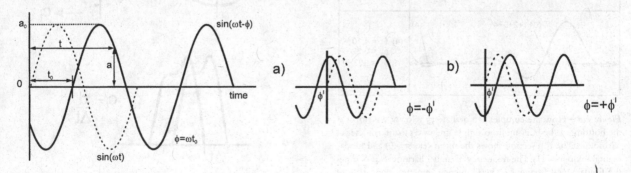

Figure 4.4 – Sine wave equation: (a) phase leads sin (ωt); (b) phase lags sin (ωt).

harmonic. To obtain the original waveform from the harmonics, each harmonic must be added to the others with the correct amplitude and phase relative to the first harmonic (Figure 4.5). The addition of each higher harmonic adds finer detail to the full complex waveform shape. In theory, the harmonic series for a complex waveform is infinite, but usually adding just the first few harmonics together produces a reasonably good likeness to the original waveform. This is because higher harmonics have much lower amplitudes so can be neglected. An example of the harmonic components for the pressure and flow waves seen in the ascending aorta is given in Appendix D.

In addition to the sinusoidal harmonic components, the waveforms have a continuous or **zero-frequency** component. This is the component that gives the **mean amplitude** of the waveform, for example the mean pressure or mean flow averaged over the cardiac cycle. By analogy with electrical theory, it is sometimes known as the DC level.

It is useful to consider the component frequencies of a waveform in this way, as complex waveforms may be dealt with and understood by considering simple sine waves.

Pulse wave velocity

The speed c_0 at which the pulse pressure wave travels peripherally down an artery is given by the **Moens–Korteweg equation**. It assumes that the vessel wall thickness h is much smaller than the vessel radius r. It also depends on the density of the fluid ρ and the stiffness or rigidity of the vessel wall E (**Young's modulus** of elasticity):

$$c_0 = \sqrt{\frac{Eh}{2r\rho}} \ (\text{m s}^{-1})$$

Moens–Korteweg Equation

The speed of the pulse pressure wave may be found by measuring the time taken for the start of the systolic pressure rise to travel between two points along a vessel (Figure 4.6).

When this measurement is made, the true speed of the pulse pressure wave c_t is found to be slightly higher than that given by the Moens–Korteweg equation because the compressibility of the vessel wall must be taken into account. This is because the wall thickness changes as it stretches. When this is done, the true speed c_t is given by:

$$c_t = 1.15 \, c_0$$

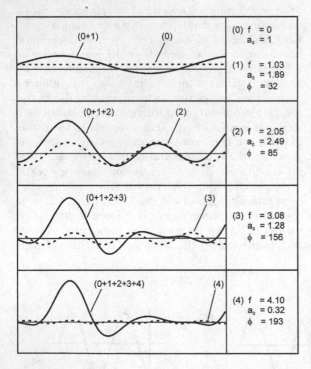

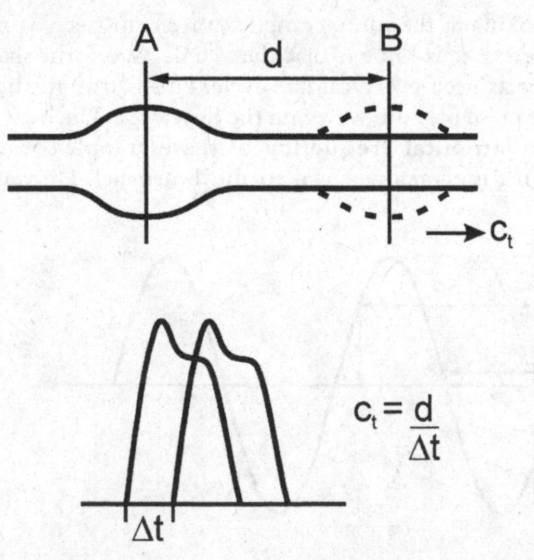

Figure 4.5 – How the complex femoral artery velocity waveform at the bottom can be built up from simple sine waves that form a set of harmonics. The top section shows the mean velocity (0) and fundamental frequency (1). The frequency of higher harmonics is N times the fundamental frequency. The frequency, amplitude and phase of each harmonic is shown (adapted from Evens and McDicken 2000).[1]

Figure 4.6 – Measurement of pulse wave velocity.

Notes from the Moens–Korteweg equation

- c_0 will increase as the radius of the vessel decreases. The speed of the pulse pressure wave will therefore increase towards the peripheral circulation.

- c_0 will increase as the elasticity (the reciprocal of rigidity, $1/E$) of the vessel wall decreases and the vessel becomes more rigid:

  - Peripheral arteries are less elastic than central arteries so c_0 will be higher in the peripheral vessels.

  - Arteriosclerosis due to disease or ageing causes the arteries to become less compliant and so c_0 will tend to be higher with age and in diseased vessels.

  - High blood pressure will preload the arterial wall compliance as described by Laplace's equation and the stress–strain diagram (Figure 3.48), and less excess movement is possible. That is, the artery is more rigid, and so c_0 will be higher.

Table 4.1 shows some typical pulse wave velocities for several arteries (Figure 4.7).

Using these values, the time taken for the pulse pressure wave to travel from the heart to the foot is ~250 ms.

Table 4.1 – Pulse wave velocity for several arteries

Ascending aorta	5.0
Thoracic aorta	5.5
Abdominal aorta	5.5
Iliac artery	8.8
Femoral artery	8.0
Radial artery	7.3
Pulmonary artery	1.7
Carotid artery	7.0

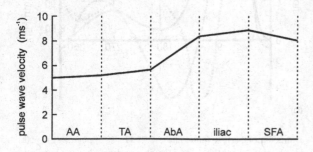

Figure 4.7 – Variation in pulse wave velocity away from the heart as measured in humans (adapted from Nichols and O'Rourke 1998).[2]

The wavelength λ_p of the pulse wave in the arterial system may also be calculated:

$$c_0 = f_{HR}\lambda_p$$

If f_{HR} = 1.2 Hz and c_0 = 5.5 ms^{-1} then λ_p = 4.6 m.

The fundamental wavelength of the pulse pressure wave is thus seen to be very much longer than the arterial tree. In fact, because of the shape of the pulse pressure wave, the whole arterial tree has dilated under the increase in pulse pressure before the pressure in the ascending aorta returns to its diastolic level.

Relationship between pulse pressure wave and flow

In the continuous flow conditions governed by Poiseuille's equation, we saw that fluid flows in response to a pressure difference along the vessel. In the case of pulsatile flow the situation is complicated by the fact that the pressure in the fluid is changing with time. Flow will still depend on pressure difference but instead of measuring a steady pressure difference over a relatively long length of tube, we need to consider the instantaneous pressure difference at a point along the tube. As the pulse pressure wave travels down the vessel, points proximal or distal to the observation point will be at a higher or lower pressure than the observation point. For example, consider the maximum pressure in the pulse pressure wave. Points along the vessel either side of the point where the maximum in the pulse pressure wave has reached must experience a lower pressure than that maximum. The steeper the fall-off in pressure away from the maximum, the greater will be the pressure difference (Figure 4.8). In other words, the instantaneous local pressure difference is the gradient of the changing pulse pressure wave. It is this **local pressure gradient** that drives the fluid along. As the gradient of the pulse pressure wave changes with time, so the fluid velocity changes and we get the **flow waveform** (Figure 4.9).

Notes on pressure and velocity waveforms

- The first thing to notice about these waveforms is that the peak in flow velocity occurs **before** the peak pressure. Although this may seem to be counter-intuitive, it is a direct consequence of the

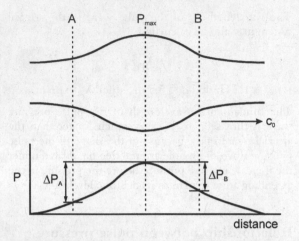

Figure 4.8 – Local pressure gradient ΔP at a point along a vessel. At A, the gradient is negative and flow will slow down; at B there is a positive gradient and flow will increase.

flow responding to the pressure gradient rather than the pressure itself. It is analogous to a surfer riding down the gradient of a wave. As the wave moves forward, the surfer continues to ride down the gradient and stays in front of the wave.

- If we observe the pulse pressure wave pass a particular point the following is seen. As long as the pressure gradient is positive the fluid will

continue to accelerate and flow will increase, as will the frictional forces within the moving fluid. After the peak pressure has passed, the pressure gradient changes sign and there will be a rapid deceleration of the fluid. The flow direction will only become negative if the pressure gradient remains negative after the fluid has been brought to rest. This is seen in arteries such as the femoral arteries where a negative-going phase in the cardiac cycle occurs. When the pressure gradient becomes positive before the fluid has been brought to rest, there will be forward flow throughout the cardiac cycle.

- The change in flow does not exactly match the change in pressure gradient but occurs slightly after it. In other words, there is a phase difference between them and the flow lags behind the pressure gradient. This is because of the effect of inertia and momentum in moving the column of fluid within the vessel. The mass of fluid cannot respond instantaneously to a very rapid change in pressure gradient. If the pressure gradient were to rise quickly and remain positive, the fluid would accelerate at a rate proportional to the pressure gradient until the frictional drag due to viscosity balanced the force to accelerate. Flow in the vessel would then be constant with a parabolic profile (see Chapter 3). Likewise, if the pressure gradient

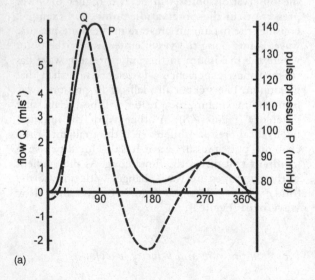

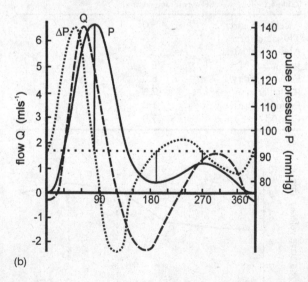

(a)   (b)

Figure 4.9 – (a) Pressure and flow waveforms recorded simultaneously in a canine femoral artery (pulse rate = 2.75 Hz, 1° of phase ≈1 ms); (b) same as (a) but with the pressure gradient curve added. This has been scaled so the similarity of shape and the phase relationship can be appreciated. Note that the points where the gradient is zero (dotted horizontal line) coincide with the maxima and minima of the pressure waveform (adapted from Nichols and O'Rourke 1998).[2]

were then to fall instantaneously to zero, the mass of fluid would continue to move forward because of its acquired momentum until viscous frictional forces slowed it down (Figure 4.10).

We may extend this argument of a phase lag in the flow due to inertia and momentum a bit further. The faster the pressure gradient changes, the greater the phase lag is likely to be as the acceleration of flow fails to keep up with the rapidly changing pressure gradient. We may also expect the phase lag to be greater in wider vessels. This is because the viscous frictional effects are particularly associated with the boundary layer near the vessel walls. In a wide vessel, the walls are further away from the centre-line, so when the fluid starts to change direction it takes longer for the viscous boundary layer to affect the bulk of the fluid. The bulk of the fluid is then initially only affected by inertial forces.

Wormersley parameter α

These features are summed up in the **Wormersley parameter** α, which, as we shall see, indicates how fluid subject to pulsatile flow behaves in a vessel. Here r is vessel radius, ρ is fluid density, μ is fluid viscosity and ω is the angular frequency ($2\pi f$) of oscillation:

$$\alpha = r\sqrt{\frac{\omega\rho}{\mu}}$$

Wormersley Parameter

The parameter is dimensionless as all units cancel.

Using a frequency of 1.2 Hz for the heart rate, we may calculate the Wormersley parameter for different vessels (Table 4.2).

The Wormersley parameter increases with increasing vessel radius and with increasing oscillatory frequency.

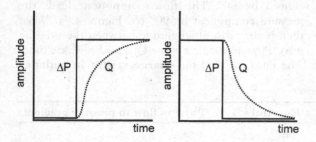

Figure 4.10 – Change in flow following a sudden increase or decrease in pressure gradient from a constant value. The solid line is pressure gradient ΔP; the dotted line is flow Q.

Table 4.2 – Wormersley parameter at resting heart rate

Ascending aorta	21
Abdominal aorta	12
External iliac artery	5.8
Superficial femoral artery	4
Posterior tibial artery	2.7
Common carotid artery	4.2

The larger α is, the greater the phase lag between pressure gradient and flow will be. This parameter therefore indicates how flow in a vessel will behave relative to the time-scale of one cycle of oscillation and the size of the vessel. In the way it indicates how the flow will behave, it is the equivalent of Reynolds number for unsteady flow.

At high values of α the magnitude of flow at each instant will be less than that predicted by Poiseuille's formula for the same pressure gradient. This is because the acceleration time will be too short to bring the fluid up to full speed before the pressure gradient changes sign and the fluid decelerates again. The flow equation for pulsatile flow at one frequency ω is shown below. For comparison, Poiseuille's equation for steady flow and the sine wave equation are also shown. This equation assumes a rigid tube, but real vessels tethered to adjacent tissue closely approximate this assumption. Here α is the Wormersley parameter, M'_{10} is a factor that itself depends on α, ω is the oscillatory frequency of the pressure wave, ϕ is the phase of the flow wave and ε'_{10} is the amount by which the flow lags the pressure gradient and depends on α. M is a constant that has the value of the maximum amplitude of the instantaneous pressure difference per unit length of vessel. (A full description of this equation and its nomenclature is given in Milnor 1982.[3]):

Pulsatile flow equation:

$$Q(t) = \left(\frac{\pi r^4}{\mu}\right)\left(\frac{M'_{10}}{a^2}\right) M \sin(\omega t - \phi - \varepsilon'_{10})$$

Poiseuille's equation:

$$Q = \frac{\pi r^4}{\mu} \cdot \frac{1}{8} \cdot \frac{\Delta P}{l}$$

Sine wave equation:

$$\alpha = \alpha_0 \sin(\omega t - \phi)$$

Figure 4.11 indicates how the phase lag between pressure gradient and flow increases, and the amplitude of flow decreases, with increasing α.

Notes:

- For $\alpha < 1$, the flow waveform will effectively match the pressure gradient waveform with no phase lag (i.e. $\varepsilon'_{10} = 0$) and no diminution in the magnitude of velocity. The amplitude constant (M'_{10}/α^2) then equals $1/8$ (0.125) as in Poiseuille's equation and the flow can be considered **quasi-steady laminar flow**, with the waveform amplitude $\frac{\pi r^4}{\mu} \cdot \frac{M}{8} = \alpha_0$ in the sine wave equation. This may be compared with the steady flow in Poiseuille's equation. This quasi-steady type flow will be seen in arteries with diameters < 1 mm.

- If α increases as a result of increasing frequency, there will be reduction in flow amplitude. This explains why the high harmonics in a waveform have low amplitudes and can usually be ignored in calculations of pulsatile flow.

- If α increases as a result of the vessel radius increasing, the r^4 term outweighs the decrease in M'_{10}/α^2 and flow increases.

- The value of α in the ascending aorta is very high (= 21). The 90° phase difference between pressure gradient and flow is emphasised by the fact that at the instant when the aortic valve opens, the pressure gradient is very large and flow in the ascending aorta is zero. At these high values of α flow is in phase with the pressure waveform.

The Pulsatile flow equation gives the flow waveform for one frequency. To determine the flow waveform produced by a pressure wave with a complex shape, the amplitude of each harmonic frequency component must be added together with the correct phase difference ($\phi - \varepsilon'_{10}$) between them (Figure 4.5).

The difference between flow calculated using Poiseuille's equation and pulsatile flow may be illustrated as follows. Assume a rigid vessel 5 mm in diameter, density of blood = 1060 kg m^{-3} and viscosity 3.5 m Pa s, then flows shown in Table 4.3 are obtained.

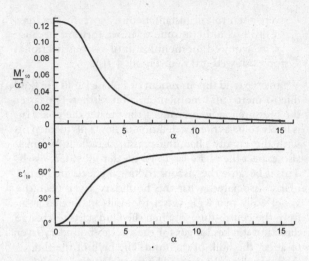

Figure 4.11 – How amplitude (M_{10}'/α^2) and phase (ϵ_{10}') of the pulsatile flow equation vary by increasing the Wormersley parameter α (adapted from Milnor 1982).[3]

Vascular impedance

For pulsatile waveforms, flow results from differences in pressure from point-to-point along the vessel. We now look at the question of how the amplitude of the flow waveform relates to the amplitude of the pressure waveform itself, rather than the pressure gradient. Consider first of all, pulsatile flow through an infinitely long, uniform elastic tube. The *shape* of the flow wave will then be the same as the *shape* of the pressure wave at any point along the tube, although there will be a phase difference between them. This is because the gradient of a sine wave is another sine wave with a phase difference of 90° (Figure 4.3a, b). So, for each harmonic component of a complex waveform, the corresponding component of the flow waveform is a harmonic of the same frequency but a different amplitude, and with phase shifted by 90°. The flow component leads the pressure component by 90° (cf. Figure 4.9a). What then is the ratio of amplitude between the pressure wave $P(t)$ and the flow wave $Q(t)$ in this elastic tube? The ratio is called the **characteristic impedance**

Table 4.3 – Comparison of steady and pulsatile flow in a 5-mm diameter tube

Flow type	Pressure gradient/frequency	Flow (ml s^{-1})	Phase of flow to pressure gradient
Steady pressure gradient	1 mmHg cm^{-1}	58	zero
Sinusoidal waveform	0.2 Hz, thus $\alpha = 0.05$	~58	phase lag << 1°
Sinusoidal waveform	2.1 Hz, thus $\alpha = 5$	14	phase lag 70°

Based on Milnor (1982).[3]

Z_0 of the tube and depends only on the properties of the tube itself, not the wave shape.

$$Z_0 = \frac{P(t)}{Q(t)} \text{ (kg m}^{-4}\text{ s}^{-1} \text{ or Pa s m}^{-3})$$

Characteristic Impedance

It can be shown that in all but the smallest arteries:

$$Z_0 = \frac{P(t)}{Q(t)} = \frac{\rho c_0}{A} = \frac{1}{A}\sqrt{\frac{\rho E h}{2r}}$$

where c_0 is the speed of sound given by the Moens–Korteweg equation.

Notes:

- The characteristic impedance as defined here, using flow, is related to the ratio of pressure to velocity by the factor of the vessel cross-sectional area, using the volume flow equation.

- The most important thing to note is that the characteristic impedance does not depend on the shape of the waveform but depends only on properties of the vessel itself. That is, the density of blood ρ, the cross-sectional area A and the speed of the pulse pressure wave c_0, involving the elastic modulus E, the wall thickness h and vessel radius r.

- In general, the characteristic impedance of arteries in the body increases towards the periphery as their radius decreases and their stiffness increases.

The term 'impedance' has been borrowed from electrical network theory, and transmission and delay line theories in particular. Electrical waveforms in these circuits behave in a similar way to pulse waves in blood vessels. Models of the arterial tree have been made using electronic circuits where, by analogy, vessel wall elasticity is modelled by capacitors, the inertial forces in blood by inductors and viscous frictional losses by resistors. Figure 4.12 shows an example of such an electrical model. Pressure is represented by voltage, and flow by current. (For a discussion of electrical analogue models, see Milnor (1982).[3])

The characteristic impedance of a vessel is a measure of the response in flow to an applied pressure. If the vessel has a small radius with stiff walls, such as is found in small peripheral arteries, the impedance will be large and the amplitude of the flow waveform for a given pressure waveform amplitude will be small. However, because the vessel has a small cross-section, the velocity $\left(v = \frac{Q}{A}\right)$ may still be quite large.

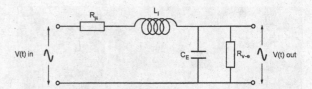

Figure 4.12 – Example of an electrical analogue model of an artery.[4] R_μ, resistance due to viscosity of blood; L_1, inertia of the blood; C_E, elastic compliance of the vessel wall; R_{v-e}, visco–elastic loss in the vessel wall.

Clinical note
Pulsatile but poor flow

When scanning the lower limb arteries of patients with narrow calcified vessels, but no discrete stenoses, the Doppler waveforms may remain pulsatile in shape to ankle level. This appearance is often seen in diabetic patients. Because the vessel is stiffened by calcification and the diameter is narrowed, the impedance of the distal tibial vessels is high. This means that for a given pressure amplitude the flow will be relatively small (Figure 4.13). This is borne out by a consideration of the volume flow in these patients compared with normals. Figure 4.13a shows an example of this in a posterior tibial artery of a diabetic. The waveform shows a nice pulsatile flow with PSV = 32 cm s^{-1}. On the other hand, the vessel lumen is very thin with calcified walls.

Using the flow equation:

$$Q = A.\text{TAV}$$

where vessel diameter = 0.14 cm, area = 0.015 cm^2, TAV = 4 cm s^{-1}, therefore flow is 3.6 ml min^{-1}.

This may be compared with a normal posterior tibial artery with PSV = 44 cm s^{-1} (Figure 4.13b).

Vessel diameter = 0.3 cm, area = 0.071 cm^2, TAV = 2.8 cm s^{-1}, therefore volume flow = 11.9 ml min^{-1}.

In these cases although the flow is pulsatile, which would normally suggest a healthy artery with good flow, the flow is in fact very low. It is the volume flow rather than velocity that determines the amount of oxygen being carried, the narrow lumen of the vessel should be recognised and the scan report should note that the flow, whilst still pulsatile, is actually very poor. Note also that measurement of blood pressure in these vessels is often quite unreliable because of the rigidity of the vessel.

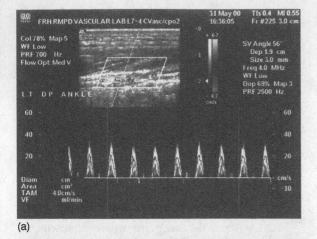

(a)

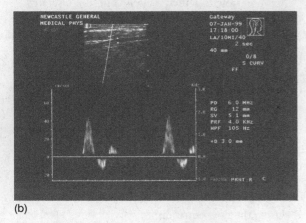

(b)

Figure 4.13 – Doppler waveforms taken from the posterior tibial artery at ankle level in (a) a diabetic patient with calcified vessel walls and a thin lumen and (b) a normal healthy artery.

In a vessel with a low characteristic impedance where the radius is large and the walls are very compliant, as is found in the proximal aorta, the amplitude of the flow waveform will be large for a given pressure waveform amplitude. However, because of the large cross-sectional area, the velocities may not be particularly high.

Characteristic impedance is analogous to the gears on a bicycle. In a low gear, equivalent to low impedance, the bicycle responds very quickly to changes in pedal pressure and acceleration is rapid. In a high gear, equivalent to a high impedance, the immediate response to changes in pedal pressure is smaller and acceleration is slower. For blood vessels, the response to changes in pressure is flow.

Impedance and fluid resistance

It is important to note that impedance is *not* a measure of the vessels resistance to flow. It is a measure of the response in flow to an applied pressure, and only applies to time-varying pressures and flows. In describing this response of flow to oscillatory pressure changes, no energy losses, such as friction due to viscosity, are considered. On the other hand, fluid resistance *is* a measure of the energy losses associated with the flow of fluid along the vessel. Fluid resistance therefore depends on the fluid viscosity and refers to the mean flow or zero frequency component.

Energy in a pulsatile wave

Travelling waves such as the pulse pressure $P(t)$ and flow $Q(t)$ waves have an energy associated with them that is transmitted along the vessel.

The mean rate of energy transmission W is given by:

$$W = P(t).Q(t) \quad (\text{J s}^{-1} \text{ or watts})$$

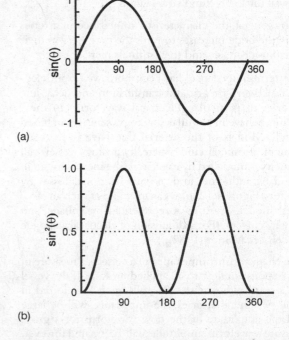

(a)

(b)

Figure 4.14 – Relationship between $\sin \theta$ and $\sin^2 \theta$: peak amplitude $a_0 = a_0^2 = 1$.

This is analogous to the expression for electrical power of voltage times current. From the definition of impedance we have:

$$Z = \frac{P(t)}{Q(t)}$$

so $W = \dfrac{P(t)^2}{Z}$ and $W = Q(t)^2 \cdot Z$

That is, the energy associated with a pulsatile wave is proportional to the square of its amplitude. For a simple sine wave variation in pressure or flow, the mean value of the amplitude is zero. However, the mean value of sine squared is not zero but half of its amplitude (Figure 4.14).

That is, transmitted energy:

$$W = \frac{1}{2}\frac{P_0^2}{Z} = \frac{1}{2}Q_0^2 \cdot Z$$

where P_0 and Q_0 are the peak amplitudes of sinusoidal pressure and flow waves. The waveforms are shown in Figure 4.15.

Figure 4.15a shows the flow $Q(t)$ produced by a simple harmonic pressure waveform $P(t)$ in which the flow leads the pressure by 90°, as previously described. In these waveforms the mean pressure and flow is zero. As shown in Chapter 3, the total fluid energy is constant but the form of energy may change from potential energy to kinetic energy and back again (the Bernoulli principle). Figure 4.15b shows that for this sinusoidal waveform when the pressure is at its maximum, the flow is zero and vice versa. In other words, the Bernoulli principle is being obeyed with energy being alternately exchanged between potential energy (pressure) and kinetic energy (flow) with each cycle.

In addition to this energy carried by the harmonic components of the pulsatile waveforms, there will also be an energy associated with the mean fluid flow. The magnitude of energy carried by the zero-frequency component is its potential and kinetic energy (see Chapter 3) where the potential energy will be the mean pressure and kinetic energy $\frac{1}{2}\rho\bar{v}^2_{\text{mean}}$.

For a cardiac output of $114\ \text{ml s}^{-1}$ ($6.8\ \text{l min}^{-1}$), the total work done by the left ventricle is 1718 mW of which

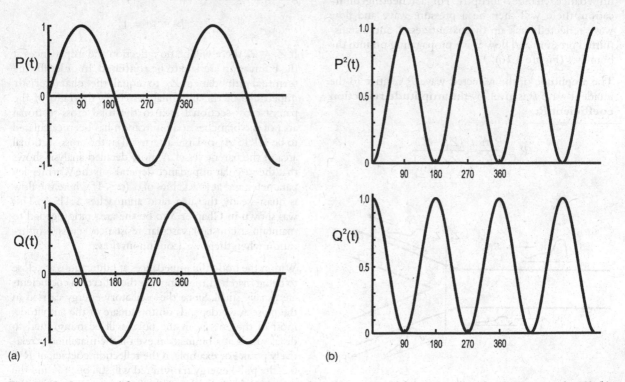

(a)   (b)

Figure 4.15 – Pressure and flow and the energy relationship between them: (a) pressure and flow waves where flow leads pressure by 90°; (b) pressure and flow energy showing that energy moves alternately between pressure and kinetic energy, as described by the Bernoulli equation.

1489 mW accounts for the zero-frequency component steady flow and 229 mW, or just 13%, is oscillatory energy. Of the total, 98% is potential energy or pressure and 2% is kinetic energy.[5]

Reflections on pulse pressure and flow waves

The characteristic impedance Z_0 describes the ratio of pulsatile pressure to flow for a vessel of infinite length. In reality, vessels in the body are relatively short before they branch. At each branching, the daughter vessels have a smaller radius and tend to be more rigid. The characteristic impedance will therefore usually change at a bifurcation, and will generally be higher in the daughter vessels. Whenever there is a change in characteristic impedance in a vessel, reflection of the pulsatile waveform will occur. This is a similar phenomenon to the reflections of sound waves seen at changes in the impedance of the medium through which they are moving. Pulse wave reflections may therefore occur at bifurcations and also at sites of disease in unbranched vessel segments where the impedance changes abruptly. For a reflecting bifurcation, there will then be a pressure wave and flow wave reflected back up the parent vessel, and a transmitted pressure and flow wave propagating on into the branches (Figure 4.16).

The amplitude of the reflected wave P_r relative to the incident wave P_i is given by the **amplitude reflection coefficient** R:

$$R = \frac{P_r(t)}{P_i(t)} = \frac{(Z_T - Z_0)}{(Z_T + Z_0)}$$

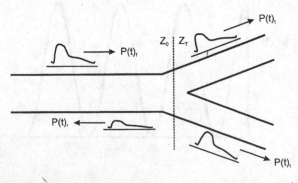

Figure 4.16 – Reflection and transmission of a pulse pressure wave at a bifurcation where there is a change in vascular impedance.

And the amplitude of the transmitted wave P_t relative to the incident wave P_i is given by the **amplitude transmission coefficient** T:

$$T = \frac{P_t(t)}{P_i(t)} = \frac{2\sqrt{Z_T Z_0}}{(Z_T + Z_0)}$$

where Z_0 is the characteristic impedance of the parent vessel and Z_T is the **terminal impedance**. For a simple bifurcation with infinitely long branches, the terminal impedance is the sum of the characteristic impedances distal to the point of reflection, that is, the two daughter vessels.

Impedances add in the same way as resistances, so for a bifurcation they add as for parallel impedances:

$$\frac{1}{Z_T} = \frac{1}{Z_1} + \frac{1}{Z_2}$$

where Z_1 and Z_2 are the characteristic impedances of the two branches.

The total energy in the reflected and transmitted waves must equal the energy in the incident wave giving the relationship:

$$T^2 + R^2 = 1$$

If $Z_T = Z_0$ there will be no reflection and impedances at the bifurcation are said to be **matched**. In order for the terminal impedance Z_T to equal the characteristic impedance of the proximal vessel Z_0, the ratio of the parent cross-sectional area to the total cross-sectional area of the branches at a bifurcation has been calculated to be 1:1.15 A_0 for large arteries. A_0 is the cross-sectional area of the parent vessel. A more detailed analysis shows that the vascular impedance depends on the Wormersley parameter and at low values of α ($\alpha < 1$) where the flow is quasi-steady, the area ratio approaches 1.41 A_0. This was shown in Chapter 3 to be the area ratio needed to maintain a constant vascular resistance across a bifurcation when there was continuous flow.

Within the body, the impedances at bifurcations are close to being matched, meaning that the reflection coefficients are usually small. Since the oscillatory energy carried in the pulse wave depends on the square of the amplitude, most of the energy in the pulse will be transmitted to distal vessels at a bifurcation even if the matching is relatively poor. For example, if the reflection coefficient $R = 0.2$, the pulse energy transmitted will still be 96% and the transmitted amplitude will be 0.98. At most junctions in the arterial tree, the reflection coefficient is < 0.2.

Reflection at an increase in vascular impedance

$$(Z_T > Z_0)$$

When $Z_T > Z_0$ the pressure wave will be reflected in-phase and the flow wave will be reflected in antiphase (i.e. 180° out of phase or inverted). Figure 4.17 shows the situation for a closed tube with a 100% reflection. Z_T is then infinite.

Consider first the pressure wave. In the case of a closed tube, the amplitude of the pressure wave adjacent to the closed end is doubled because the reflected wave is in-phase with the incident pressure wave and adds to it. At

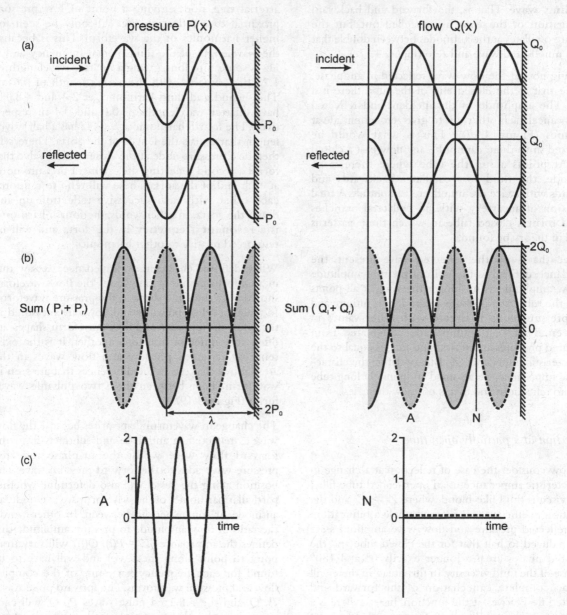

Figure 4.17 – Pressure and flow waveforms reflected at a closed-end tube with no energy losses: (a) incident and reflected waveforms along the tube at an instant in time: note that the pressure waveform is reflected in-phase and the flow waveform is reflected in antiphase; (b) peak amplitude envelope along the tube of the sum of incident and reflected waves forms a standing wave pattern which shows the presence of nodes N and antinodes A; (c) time-varying waveforms occurring at an antinode A and node N.

a distance of $\lambda/4$ from the end, the amplitude of oscillation will be zero and there is a pressure node. At a distance of $\lambda/2$ there will again be a doubling of amplitude forming an antinode, and so on up the tube. This summation of a forward-moving incident pressure wave and backward-moving reflected pressure wave forms a pattern of nodes and antinodes known as a **standing wave**. That is, the forward and backward propagation of the wave is cancelled out, but the pressure oscillates at the antinodes between double that of the unreflected wave and zero (Figure 4.17c).

Looking now at the flow wave reflected in antiphase, we see that at the closed end of the tube there is a node. The amplitude of the incident and reflected waves cancel each other out to give zero amplitude at all times (Figure 4.17c). This is what would be expected since there cannot be any flow past a closed end. At points along the tube where there is an antinode, the fluid just oscillates backwards and forwards with twice the unreflected amplitude. A total occlusion of an artery with no collateral branches would form a closed tube in which these patterns could in theory be found.

Notice that with the reflected wave present, the impedance, defined as the ratio of pressure amplitude to flow amplitude, is no longer the same at all points along the tube. At a pressure antinode it is infinite and at a pressure node it is zero with other values in between. That is, the impedance calculated from measured pressures and flows is no longer equal to the characteristic impedance Z_0. But, to define the characteristic impedance, we assumed an infinitely long tube with no reflections and that is not now the case.

Reflection at a partially open tube

We now consider the case of reflection at a change in characteristic impedance in an open-ended tube filled with viscous fluid like blood, where $Z_T > Z_0$ and the reflection coefficient is 0.5, for example a bifurcation. The reflected pressure and flow wave amplitudes are then reduced to half that for the closed tube and the reflected phases are no longer exactly 0° and 180° because of the fluid viscosity. In this situation there will not be complete cancellation of the forward and reflected flow waves at the junction. Instead there is a reduction in the amplitude of the forward flow wave compared with a perfectly matched change in impedance ($Z_T = Z_0$), and for the pressure wave there is only a **partial standing wave** (Figure 4.18).

Reflections at the aortic bifurcation into the abdominal aorta are of this type. The amplitude reflection coefficient at the aortic bifurcation is ~0.16 in man. The increase in pressure caused by the pressure wave being reflected in-phase is thought to be a contributory factor in the development of abdominal aortic aneurysms. Within the human arterial tree, nodes giving a point of low pressure proximal to a reflecting site will only be seen for higher harmonics of the waveform. This is because the wavelength of the fundamental frequency at 1.2 Hz is some 5 m long giving a quarter wavelength of 1.25 m compared with the aorta's length of 0.6 m. The second and third harmonics at 2.4 and 4.8 Hz have quarter wavelengths of 0.6 and 0.4 m respectively. The fourth harmonic at 9.6 Hz has a half wavelength that equals the length of the aorta. There will then be a pressure node at the closed aortic valve that forms a second reflecting site, giving a pressure node at each end of the aorta. These will tend to reinforce each other with each successive reflection up and down the aorta. In other words, the fourth harmonic is a **resonant frequency** in the aorta and will be reinforced relative to other harmonics.

When defining characteristic impedance, we saw that in a uniform infinitely long vessel, the flow waveform should have the same shape as the pressure waveform. In practice, when pressures and flows are measured in the body, the pressure and flow waveform shapes are often very different from one another. It is the existence of reflected pressure and flow waves in the arterial tree that causes the differences that are seen in waveform shape between these two pulsatile waveforms (Figure 4.19).

The change in waveform shape arises because the flow wave is reflected in antiphase and subtracts from the forward flow wave whilst the in-phase reflected pressure wave adds to the forward pressure wave. The position along the vessel will also determine whether particular harmonics of the waveform are at a node, an antinode or somewhere in between. In other words, the ratio of flow amplitude to pressure amplitude that defines the impedance ($Z = P(t)/Q(t)$) will vary from point to point along the vessel and will have to be found for each frequency harmonic of the complex flow and pressure waveforms. The forward pulse waves P_i, Q_i and the reflected pulse waves P_r, Q_r will each depend on the characteristic impedance of the vessel Z_0, but the impedance calculated from the measured pulse waves $P_m = P_i + P_r$ and $Q_m = Q_i - Q_r$ will vary along the vessel and vary with frequency as described.

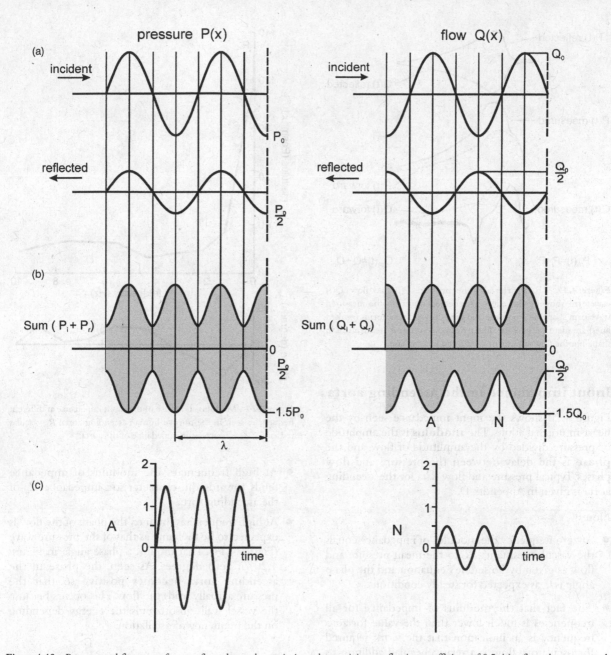

Figure 4.18 – Pressure and flow waveforms reflected at a change in impedance giving a reflection coefficient of 0.5: (a) reflected pressure and flow waves have an amplitude 50% that of the incident wave; (b) sum of the incident and reflected waves form a partial standing wave in which the peak envelope varies in amplitude along the tube between 0.5 and 1.5; (c) this is shown in the time-varying waveforms occurring at an antinode A and node N.

This impedance calculated from the actual pulse waves is known as the **input impedance** and is the impedance seen by the vessel distal to the point of measurement. At a bifurcation the input impedance is

the same as the terminal impedance Z_T described before when discussing reflected pulse waves. At the aortic root the input impedance is the impedance of the whole systemic circulation as seen by the heart.

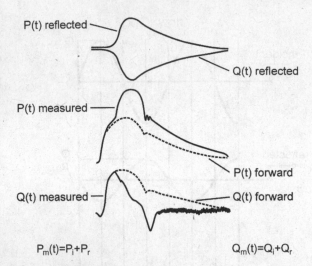

$$P_m(t)=P_i+P_r \qquad\qquad Q_m(t)=Q_i+Q_r$$

Figure 4.19 – Real arterial pulse pressure $P(t)$ and flow $Q(t)$ waveform showing the effect of reflected waves on the measured waveform shape. The pressure and flow-forward waveforms (broken lines) are identical in shape. The reflected waveforms are identical in shape but the flow waveform is reflected in antiphase.[6]

Input impedance in the ascending aorta

Figure 4.20 shows the input impedance seen by the heart in normal adults. The **modulus** is the amplitude of pressure divided by the amplitude of flow, and the **phase** is the delay between the pressure and flow phases. Typical pressure and flow data for the ascending aorta is given in Appendix D.

Notes:

- At zero frequency the modulus of impedance equals the vascular resistance R_f to the mean pressure and flow as given by Poiseuille's equation and the phase angle is 0, as expected for steady conditions.

- The fact that the modulus of impedance for all frequencies is much lower than the value for zero frequency is an indication that the work required for oscillatory flow is a relatively small addition to the work required for continuous flow.

- At low frequencies the phase difference between pressure and flow tends towards −90° as expected, with flow leading pressure.

- Between 2 and 6 Hz the modulus of impedance is low. This has important implications for the work required of the heart to pump blood round the circulation (see Chapter 5).

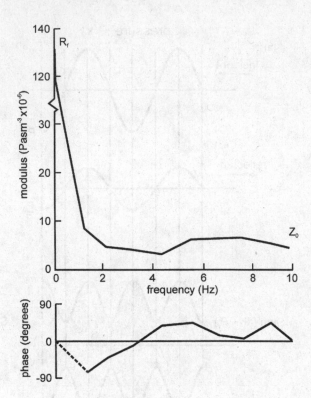

Figure 4.20 – Modulus and phase of the input impedance at different frequencies seen in the normal human ascending aorta. R_f, vascular resistance; Z_0, characteristic impedance of the aorta.[5]

- At high frequencies the modulus of impedance tends towards the characteristic impedance Z_0 of the ascending aorta.

- At high frequencies (high α) the phase of the flow is expected to be the same as that of the pressure wave (Figure 4.11). That implies a phase angle in Figure 4.20 of zero degrees. As seen, the phase in the ascending aorta becomes positive so that the pressure actually leads the flow. This occurs because the vessel walls absorb pulsatile energy depending on the frequency of oscillation.

Attenuation of the pulse pressure wave

We have seen that the energy associated with the oscillatory components of the pulse wave is proportional to the square of the pulse amplitude. As the pulse wave travels along the vessel, work must be done to overcome frictional forces. These arise both in the fluid due to viscosity, and in stretching the vessel walls which are not perfectly elastic but have viscous-type of losses associated with their movement. In the walls they are known as **visco–elastic**

losses and they depend on the frequency of oscillation. Dissipating energy to these viscous and visco-elastic losses causes the amplitude of the pulse pressure wave to be attenuated as it travels along the vessel.

As Figure 4.21 shows, blood viscosity only contributes 25–30% of the total attenuation of the pulsitility. The rest is due to losses in the visco-elastic vessel wall. Both forward-moving and reflected pulse waves will be attenuated by these mechanisms. The attenuation increases with the frequency of the wave, so high harmonics will be more strongly attenuated than low ones. This leads to a change in waveform shape as the pulse travels down the arterial tree whereby the lower frequency components predominate and the waveform becomes more rounded and damped. This becomes more significant in the smaller arteries of < 1 mm diameter.

Vessel taper and pulse amplification

Working in the opposite sense to attenuation is the fact that the radius decreases and the elasticity of the arterial walls decreases towards the peripheral circulation. These features are respectively known as **radial taper** and **elastic taper**. Their effect in increasing the speed of propagation of the pulse pressure wave has already been noted. They also produce a gradual increase in the characteristic impedance along an unbranched length of vessel.

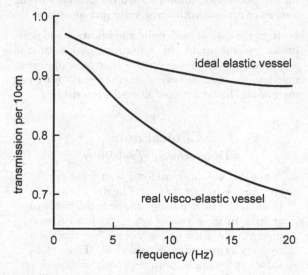

Figure 4.21 – Transmission per 10 cm of a pulse pressure wave in the aorta. The upper curve shows the theoretical values for a vessel with perfectly elastic walls. The only attenuation is then due to fluid viscosity. The lower curve shows measured values made in a real aorta and includes the visco-elastic losses in the vessel walls. These arise mainly from the smooth muscle component in the walls.[2]

This gradual increase in impedance along a vessel may be considered to be a series of small steps in which all the energy in the pulse wave is transmitted and none is reflected (Figure 4.22). The flow of energy W in a pressure wave is related to the square of the pressure amplitude P_0 and to the impedance Z, so:

$$P_0 = \text{constant.} \sqrt{Z}$$

Therefore if the impedance Z gradually increases, the pulse pressure amplitude will increase. That is, there is an amplification of the pulse pressure wave as it travels down the vessel. Similarly, energy in the flow wave $Q(t)$ is proportional to $1/\sqrt{Z}$ and so the amplitude of the flow wave will decrease:

$$Q(t) = \text{constant}/\sqrt{Z}$$

This phenomenon is seen in vessels down to 1–2 mm diameter (Figure 4.23).

Non-linear effects on wave shape

In addition to the effects of attenuation and amplification from radial and elastic taper, non-linear effects can alter the waveform shape. The effect of attenuation is to reduce the high-frequency components more than the low ones. The effect of non-linearity is the opposite, to increase the pulsatility of the waveform by moving energy from low-frequency harmonics into higher frequency ones. The result of this is to increase the steepness of the systolic rise so that the peak moves towards the start of systole. This is similar to the steepening of sea waves as they approach the shore. There are two causes of this non-linear effect.

The first cause is the fact that the stress–strain curve for arterial walls is non-linear (Figures 3.47 and 3.48).

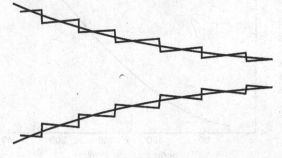

Figure 4.22 – A gradually tapering tube can be represented by a succession of small discontinuities, each of which gives rise to negligible reflection.[7]

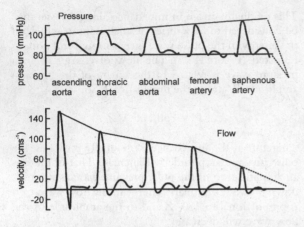

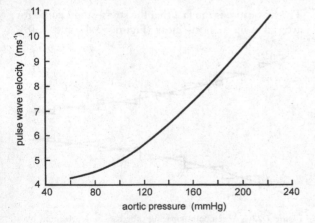

Figure 4.23 – Pressure and velocity waveforms in arteries as they travel away from the heart adapted from measurements made in dogs. The waveforms show the effects of amplification of the pressure wave due to radial and elastic taper as well as those due to reflection.[2]

Therefore, as pressure increases during systole, the vessel wall becomes more rigid and the pulse wave velocity increases causing a steepening in the acceleration phase of the systolic peak. Figure 4.24 shows this effect in the canine aorta.

The second cause occurs in the presence of reflected waves. The speed of the pulse wave (c_0) should really be measured relative to the local fluid speed v rather than the stationary vessel wall. This means that the forward wave speed is $(c + v)$ and the reflected wave speed is $(c - v)$ (Figure 4.25). This combination of speeds will also tend to steepen the acceleration phase of the systolic peak.

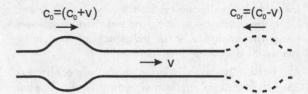

Figure 4.25 – Forward and reflected pulse wave velocity relative to the velocity of blood flow.

These mechanisms are not usually apparent in normal vessels. However, they will be effective where the arteries are abnormally distensible, giving low pulse wave velocity, or when the pulse amplitude is very large so that fluid velocity and the increase in systolic pressure is large. For example, this phenomenon may be seen in the pulmonary arteries which are more distensible with a larger relative pressure change than the systemic arteries. The presence of aortic valve regurgitation causes the pulse pressure variation in the aorta to increase greatly as the heart responds by enlarging and increasing the stroke volume in an attempt to maintain the peripheral circulation.

In the arterial tree the steepening of the systolic peak does not appear to become infinite and reach a point of 'shock', where as, in the case of a sea wave, the wave breaks with a large energy loss. However, the formation of a shock wave has been suggested as the mechanism for the 'pistol-shot' sounds sometimes observed in the arteries of patients with aortic valve incompetence.

Note: in the case of both pulse amplification and non-linear enhancement of pulsatility, although the amplitude of the pressure wave increases, the mean fluid pressure must decrease along the vessel. Otherwise there would be no net flow along the arterial tree.

Clinical note
Distal recovery of pulsatility

A pulsatile velocity waveform with a fast systolic rise time is sometimes seen in the distal tibial vessels when there is major disease in the proximal arteries. In these cases a poor waveform is seen immediately distal to the disease, but there is a recovery of pulsatility at ankle level. Figure 4.26 shows an example from a patient with severe occlusive disease in the aorto–iliac segment. The proximal superficial femoral artery shows a damped waveform (a). In contrast, the waveform from the posterior tibial artery at ankle level shows a reasonably pulsatile waveform (b), although PSV

Figure 4.24 – Variation in pulse wave velocity with aortic pressure measured in the canine aorta (adapted from Histand and Ankler 1973).[8]

is only 20 cm s^{-1} (normally > 40 cm s^{-1}). This is due to the amplification of the pulse pressure wave by radial and elastic taper of the vessels and by reflection and non-linear phenomena. In this situation care needs to be taken in reporting the findings so as not to give a misleading impression that underestimates the severity of the proximal disease. Although the distal waveform appears pulsatile in shape, the velocities will be low and the volume flow will actually be very poor. Rather than describe the distal flow as pulsatile, it is better to indicate that the flow appears poor (based on the velocities) but that the vessels are patent, indicating a good run-off.

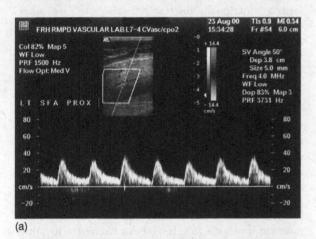

(a)

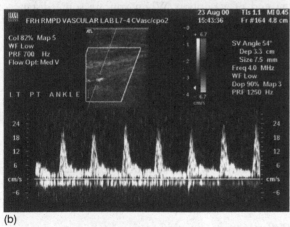

(b)

Figure 4.26 – Doppler waveforms illustrating recovery of pulsatility: (a) damped waveform seen in the superficial femoral artery distal to severe iliac stenoses; (b) waveform in the posterior tibial artery of the same patient showing a pulsatile waveform but with poor flow.

Sites of pulse wave reflection

We know that there must be significant sites of reflection of the pulse wave along the arterial tree because the shape of the flow waveform is different to that of the pressure waveform. However, the question of determining where these reflections occur is complicated by the fact that there are so many branches within the arterial tree and the low-frequency harmonics have a wavelength that is much longer than any branch. Three approaches could be used. The first is to look for individual bifurcations where there is a significant change in vascular impedance that will produce reflections. The second is to look for nodes in any partial standing waves in the pressure waveforms and calculate where the reflection is occurring downstream from the node. The third is to look at the timing of the notch or incisura on the antegrade wave caused by a reflected wave to determine where the reflection causing it is originating.

The third method is the one we shall use. Reflection at a bifurcation with $Z_T > Z_0$ will produce a reflected flow wave in antiphase to the forward flow wave. The effect of this reflection is to produce a notch on the envelope of the forward flow wave, as may be seen on some Doppler waveforms (Figure 4.27). The way this notch relates to the pressure and flow waves is shown in Figure 4.19.

The time at which this notch occurs after the start of systole depends on the time taken for the pulse wave to travel out to the reflecting site and back up the artery to the point of observation. For a single reflecting bifurcation the notch will occur at a time Δt_p after the incident wave has passed by the point of observation.

$$\Delta t_p = \frac{2L_z}{c_0}$$

where c_0 is pulse wave velocity and L_z is the distance downstream of the reflecting site.

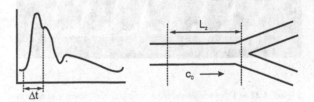

Figure 4.27 – Parameters used in the calculation of the notch position due to a reflected wave.

Clinical note
Secondary peak in femoral arteries

The normal waveform seen in common femoral and proximal superficial femoral arteries is the triphasic waveform seen in Figure 4.28a. The waveform shown in (b) where there is a secondary peak or 'knee' on the descending slope of the systolic peak is sometimes seen at these sites. This is due to a reflected wave from distal disease. It may be due to a localised tight stenosis or to generalised narrowing of the SFA and distal vessels. If this waveform is seen, the vessel should be thoroughly examined for cause.

Reflection from multiple branches

In the real arterial tree, because the pulse wave velocity is so high (5–8 m s^{-1}), reflections from multiple branchings will overlap one another. Therefore, we should really consider reflections from the whole arterial tree rather than at individual bifurcations (Figure 4.29).

Using models of the arterial tree and calculating the effect of reflections from all the branchings, it is found that all

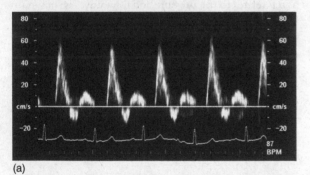

(a)

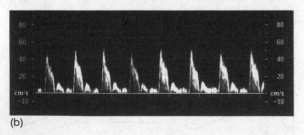

(b)

Figure 4.28 – Doppler waveforms from (a) the normal common femoral artery (CFA) and (b) the CFA in a patient with occlusion of the superficial femoral artery at mid-thigh showing a secondary peak due to a reflected wave.

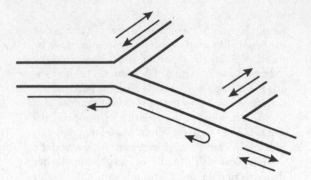

Figure 4.29 – Multiple reflections from multiple branchings.

the distal reflections from many sites combine together to form a 'functionally discrete reflecting site'.[2] In other words, they behave as though there was a single reflecting site some distance L_z away from the point of observation. Rearranging the last equation, that distance is given by:

$$L_z = c_0 \frac{\Delta t_p}{2}$$

The functional sites of reflection calculated in this way are usually found to be close to the next major vessel junction. In the aorta it is near the aortic bifurcation, in the femoral artery it is near the distal popliteal branches and in the subclavian artery it is just above the elbow. Because the reflection is caused by all the junctions distally and not just the next junction down the line, it has been likened to locating the end of a rainbow. When you are some distance away, you can say where it is, but as you move towards it, it keeps receding from you and you never actually reach it. The largest contribution to the reflected component in fact comes from the high impedance terminal vessels of the arterial tree – the arterioles. This fact is demonstrated when the peripheral vasculature is dilated, for instance following vigorous exercise or by using vasodilator drugs. When the arterioles are dilated, the impedance mismatch of the terminal junctions is reduced and the reflected pressure and flow wave seen in the proximal arteries is reduced or abolished altogether (Figure 4.31b).

Reflections at aortic bifurcation

If we look at the pressure and flow waves in the aorta given in Figure 4.31, we can see the effects of the functional reflecting site at the aortic bifurcation.

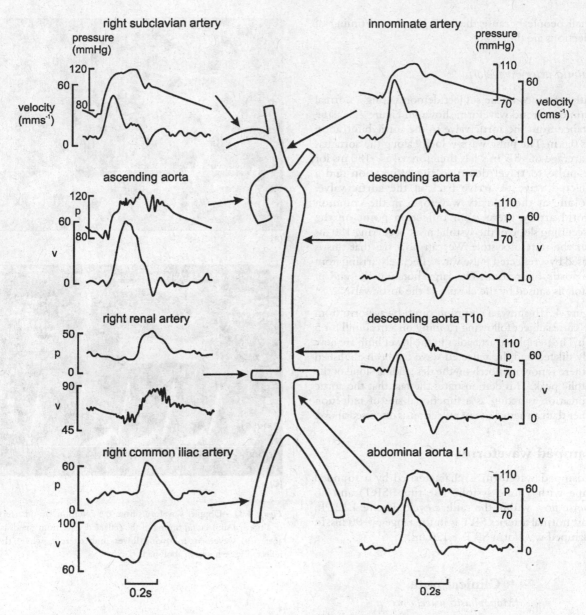

Figure 4.30 – Pressure and velocity waveforms around the central arteries recorded in a human subject undergoing diagnostic cardiac catheterisation and recorded with an electromagnetic flowmeter.[9]

Notice that the inflection point in the waveforms for the aorta occur later in the cardiac cycle the higher up the aorta one looks. For the pressure wave, the in-phase reflection results in an elongation of the systolic, high-pressure region of the wave. The effect of such reflected pressure waves in the aorta together with the elastic tapering of the aorta is important to the functioning of the heart. By lengthening the pulse pressure wave in the ascending aorta, they reduce the impedance seen by the heart and improve its efficiency as a pump (see Chapter 5).

The waveform shape will also vary with age and disease since attendant changes in arterial wall stiffness and arterial diameter alter the pulse wave speed and impedance of the arteries. Children and adults of small stature will have somewhat different waveform shapes to tall people because the path length and timing of reflections are different.

Carotid artery waveform

With reference to the subject demonstrating a normal common carotid waveform shown in Figure 4.31a, the distance from the aortic valve to the aortic bifurcation was 0.6 m. The pulse wave velocity along the aorta has an average of ~5.5 m s⁻¹. It therefore takes ~180 ms for the pulse to travel down to the bifurcation and a reflected wave to arrive back at the aortic valve. Looking at the velocity waveform in the common carotid artery, there is an inflection point on the descending slope of the systolic peak occurring 180 ms after the start of systole. We can now see that this is caused by a reflected pulse wave effectively arising from the aortic bifurcation. The large notch at the end of systole is caused by the closure of the aortic valve.

Figure 4.31b shows a common carotid waveform from the same subject following running on a treadmill for 5 min. The peripheral arterioles in the lower limb are now fully dilated and the reflected wave has been abolished so there is now no notch on the descending slope of the systolic peak. This demonstrates the fact that the aortic bifurcation is acting as a functional site of reflection rather than an actual site of reflection as discussed above.

Damped waveforms

A damped waveform is characterised by a rounded shape with a long systolic rise time (SRT) and no reverse flow within the cardiac cycle (Figure 4.32). In most normal arteries SRT is in the range 60–90 ms. In a damped waveform SRT > 120 ms.

Clinical note
'Monophasic' waveforms

In reporting waveforms, those with no reverse component of flow, such as damped waveforms, are sometimes described as monophasic. However, the normal carotid artery waveform is also monophasic, but with a fast systolic rise time and a window under the systolic peak it is a pulsatile waveform. Therefore, the term 'monophasic' on its own can be ambiguous in describing the type of flow seen. The terms 'pulsatile' and 'damped' are far more informative in describing the quality of flow.

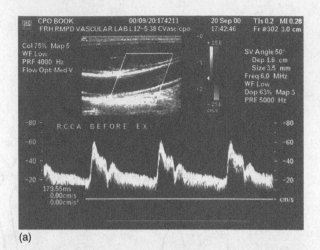

(a)

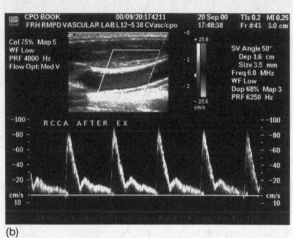

(b)

Figure 4.31 – Doppler waveforms from the common carotid artery of a normal subject: (a) timing of the reflected wave from the distal aorta; (b) waveform following lower limb exercise where the reflected wave has been abolished.

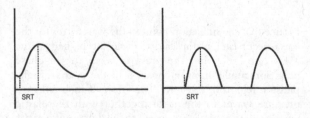

Figure 4.32 – Damped waveforms. Systolic rise time > 120 ms.

There are a number of causes of waveform damping:

- Towards the periphery of the arterial tree, in vessels < 1 mm in diameter, the waveforms become more damped. This is because there is increased attenuation of the higher frequency harmonics of the pulse waveform as the Wormersley parameter α decreases. The effect of removing the high-frequency components of the waveform is for the waveform shape to lose detailed structure including a less rapidly changing pressure or velocity. In other words, the waveform becomes more damped in appearance with the fundamental cardiac frequency predominating. Similar damping of flow may also be seen in large arteries where there is generalised narrowing rather than discrete stenosis.

- Distal to a tight stenosis the waveform may become damped. The resistance of the stenosis and the compliance of the distal vessel together act as a low-pass filter removing the high-frequency components[10]. In this situation the degree of stenosis limits the volume flow as shown in Chapter 3. The stenosis is analogous to the electrical circuit shown in Figure 4.33.

- In vessels where flow is high and there is turbulence throughout most of the cardiac cycle, the distal waveform shape will be damped. The presence of turbulence indicates that the Reynolds number is high. Flow is then unlikely to increase significantly with any further physiological change other than an increase in heart rate. In these circumstances the vessel may be considered to be carrying its **maximal flow** with the vessel's own intrinsic diameter being the limiting factor.

This sort of flow is sometimes seen in vessels acting as collaterals when other major vessels are occluded. For example, damped flow may be seen in the vertebral arteries when one or both internal carotid arteries are occluded. It may also be seen in vessels carrying a large flow following vigorous exercise of the muscles in the peripheral vascular bed or in arteries supplying arterio-venous malformations.

Note: a qualitative indication of the volume flow in an artery may be made by comparing the waveform shape, vessel diameter and peak systolic velocity.

Clinical note
Damped waveform in a normal artery

The observation of a damped waveform in an otherwise apparently normal artery may be due to either proximal disease or that the artery is acting as a collateral and is carrying an abnormally high flow. Care should be taken to determine the cause. In either case the artery is probably carrying its maximal flow whether that flow is limited by a stenosis or by the artery's own intrinsic diameter. A useful measure of whether a waveform is significantly damped is the systolic rise time (SRT). In normal arteries SRT is usually < 100 ms. If SRT $\geq$ 120 ms and the waveform has a monophasic shape, it may be said to be damped.

Figure 4.34 shows a damped waveform from the vertebral artery of a patient with an ipsilateral internal carotid artery occlusion. The vertebral diameter = 0.29 cm and TAV = 20 cm s^{-1}, giving a flow = 79 ml min^{-1}. This vertebral artery is probably carrying its maximal flow.

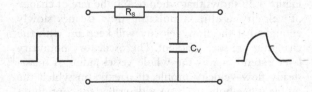

Figure 4.33 – Effect of a low-pass filter on a square waveform. R_s, resistance of a stenosis; C_v, compliance of the distal vessel.

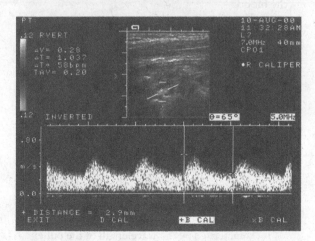

Figure 4.34 – Doppler waveform from a vertebral artery acting as collateral in a patient with an ipsilateral internal carotid occlusion. Flow is damped and maximal.

Velocity profiles

For pulsatile flow, the relationship between the motion of the central core fluid to the viscous boundary layer is most clearly seen in the way the velocity profile changes with time. Fluid is accelerated by the instantaneous pressure gradient along the vessel and acquires momentum as it does so. As the fluid moves along the vessel, viscous forces develop adjacent to the vessel walls and a viscous boundary layer begins to move in from the walls towards the centre line by **viscous diffusion**. The longer the fluid flows in one direction, the greater the thickness of the boundary layer that will develop. The degree to which the boundary layer affects the velocity profile will therefore depend on the frequency of oscillation and the diameter of the vessel. The frequency determines the time available for the boundary layer to develop and the vessel diameter determines how thick the boundary layer must grow to affect all of the fluid. We have already seen that these factors are summarised in the Wormersley parameter α.

> ### Technical note
> #### *Comparison of the Wormersley parameter α with an entrance boundary layer*
>
> The Wormersley parameter α may be compared with the equation given for the development of the boundary layer δ under 'Entrance effects' in Chapter 3.[11] The boundary layer thickness δ depends on distance x from the vessel entrance and the velocity v, viscosity μ and density ρ of the blood:
>
> Entrance boundary layer:
>
> $$\delta \propto \sqrt{\frac{x}{v} \cdot \frac{\mu}{\rho}}$$
>
> Wormersley parameter:
>
> $$\alpha = r \sqrt{\frac{\omega \rho}{\mu}}$$
>
> Consider two cases for a simple sinusoidal pulse wave.
>
> 1 As flow begins to accelerate at the start of a new cycle, the length of tube along which the boundary layer can grow before the cycle ends is characterised by the wavelength of the pulse:
>
> $$c_0 = f.\lambda$$

or in terms of angular frequency ω:

$$c_0 = \frac{\omega.\lambda}{2\pi}$$

Substituting c_0 for velocity v and wavelength λ for distance x in the entrance boundary layer equation:

$$\delta \propto \sqrt{\frac{\lambda}{c_0} \cdot \frac{\mu}{\rho}} \propto \sqrt{\frac{\mu}{\omega \rho}} = \delta_{osc}$$

now substituting this into the Wormersley parameter:

$$\alpha = \frac{r}{\delta_{ocs}}$$

we see that the parameter α is the ratio of tube radius r to the oscillatory boundary layer thickness δ_{osc}.

2 Using $v = x/t$ in the entrance boundary layer equation, the time taken for the boundary layer δ to fill the tube is:

$$\delta = r \propto \sqrt{t_\delta \cdot \frac{\mu}{\rho}} \quad so \quad \frac{\rho}{\mu} \propto \frac{t_\delta}{r^2}$$

substituting this into the Wormersley parameter:

$$\alpha^2 = \omega t_\delta = \frac{t_\delta}{T}$$

and we see that α^2 is the ratio of the viscous diffusion time to the period of oscillation T.

Figure 4.35 shows the way the velocity profile varies across one cycle of oscillation for four values of α. The pressure pulse shape in this example is a pure sine wave.

In each case the thing that characterises the velocity profiles seen is not the frequency of oscillation or the vessel diameter but the Wormersley parameter α. If the vessel width were increased and the frequency of oscillation decreased such that α remained the same, the same set of velocity profiles would be obtained.

Figure 4.35 shows that when $\alpha < 1$, the rate of change of velocity within a pulsatile flow occurs slowly enough that the flow velocity will keep up with the changing pressure gradient. The oscillatory boundary layer extends across the whole vessel radius. A quasi-steady flow–velocity profile then exists in which the profile is parabolic in shape as described for continuous Poiseuille flow. Within the normal arterial tree, this situation will be seen in vessels < 1.4 mm diameter.

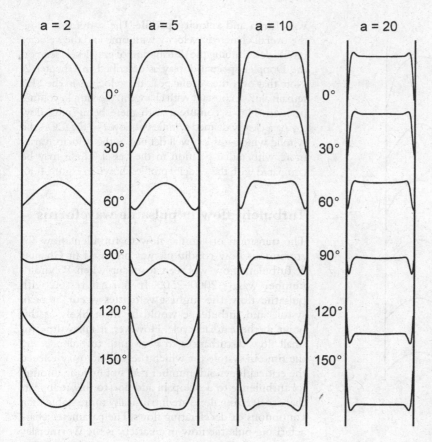

a = 2   a = 5   a = 10   a = 20

0°

30°

60°

90°

120°

150°

Figure 4.35 – Velocity profiles for sinusoidal flow for various Wormersley parameters α. The profiles have been drawn so that the maximum velocity at zero degrees is the same in all cases. In reality, the amplitude of oscillation will be smaller at higher α's. Only half the cycle has been shown as the other half is identical. Velocity is always zero at the vessel wall.[1]

The velocity profiles for real pressure and flow waveforms may be calculated by adding the velocity profiles for each harmonic of the complex waveform with the correct amplitude and phase. Two examples, common femoral and common carotid arteries, are shown in Figure 4.36.

Notes:

- During systole the velocity profile is flattened as the fluid accelerates from a low velocity. In the case of an artery such as the aorta or SFA, the velocity accelerates from zero. This situation is similar to that described for 'Entrance effects' in Chapter 3. The effect of a flattened velocity profile (plug flow) is to give a window on the Doppler spectrum. This window is seen under the acceleration phase of the systolic peak and is more prominent when the end-diastolic flow is zero.

- In the case of an artery with continuous forward flow throughout the cardiac cycle, such as the common carotid artery (CCA), the velocity profiles are seen to have a quasi-parabolic shape throughout. This signifies a large zero frequency component flowing into a low peripheral resistance.

- At some points within the cardiac cycle there may be flow in both directions simultaneously. At these times the boundary layer has responded quickly to a change in the direction of the pressure gradient whilst the momentum of the core flow still carries it forward. This will show on the Doppler spectrum as bi-directional flow at the phase when it occurs (Figure 4.37). Bi-directional flow on a Doppler spectrum will also be seen when there are secondary rotational flows and when there is turbulence creating vortices.

- In some vessels the flow at end-diastole is stationary or quasi-stationary.

Direct measurements of the time-varying velocity profile may be made by using pulsed Doppler ultrasound with a very narrow range gate. Velocity waveforms are obtained from a number of steps across the vessel lumen and these are then redrawn to show the way the velocity profile changes over the cardiac cycle. Figure 4.38 shows the change in the Doppler waveform for steps across the CCA (a) and superficial femoral artery SFA (b). Figure 4.38 shows in detail the relationship between the **velocity**

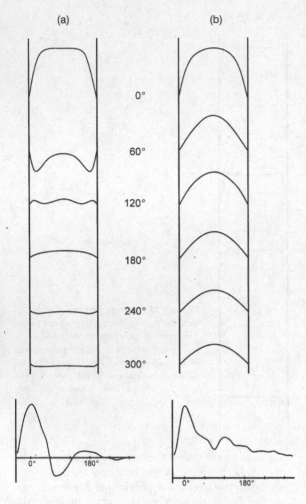

Figure 4.36 – Velocity profiles for (a) the common femoral artery and (b) the common carotid artery. The velocity waveforms are shown so that the phase position of the profiles can be identified.[1]

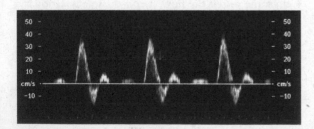

Figure 4.37 – Doppler waveform from the common femoral artery showing bi-directional flow at one part of the cycle.

waveform and **velocity profile**. The waveform being the overall change in velocity with time and the velocity profile determining the distribution of grey levels seen on the Doppler spectral display as described in Chapter 2. Note that over the systolic peak the velocities in the SFA remain almost constant with change in the sample volume position. This is consistent with there being plug flow giving a clearly defined systolic window. For the CCA the systolic window is less well defined as the velocity varies more with radial position in the vessel. These may be compared with the velocity profiles shown in Figure 4.36.

Turbulent flow in pulsatile waveforms

The transition of laminar flow to turbulent flow for continuous flow conditions was discussed in Chapter 3. Turbulent flow was seen to occur when Reynolds number was > 2000–2500. In normal vessels with pulsatile flow, the highest velocities occur at peak systole and turbulence would be most likely at this point in the cardiac cycle. However, it takes time for small flow disturbances to grow into turbulence and the time in systole for which the velocity may exceed the critical Reynolds number may not be long enough for turbulence to develop. In addition to this, it appears that accelerating flows are intrinsically more stable than continuous or decelerating flows. The parameter characterising pulsatile flow in an artery is the Wormersley parameter α. Experimental measurements have shown that the Reynolds number calculated for the peak systolic velocity may be related to α to give a critical peak Reynolds number Re_{pc}.

$$Re_{pc} > 200\,\alpha$$

The critical peak Reynolds number for some vessels is given in Table 4.4.

Turbulence is sometimes observed in the normal thoracic aorta at rest where it begins at peak systole, and having developed it continues through the decelerating phase of the peak. Where there is turbulent flow at a pipe entrance, the entrance length is shortened because there is greater

Table 4.4 – Critical peak Reynolds number for some vessels

	α	PSV (m s^{-1})	Re_{PSV}	Re_{PSV}/α
Ascending aorta	21	1.12	9400	448
Abdominal aorta	12	0.75	3600	300
Femoral artery	4.0	0.60	860	215
Carotid artery	4.2	0.80	1700	405

(a)

(b)

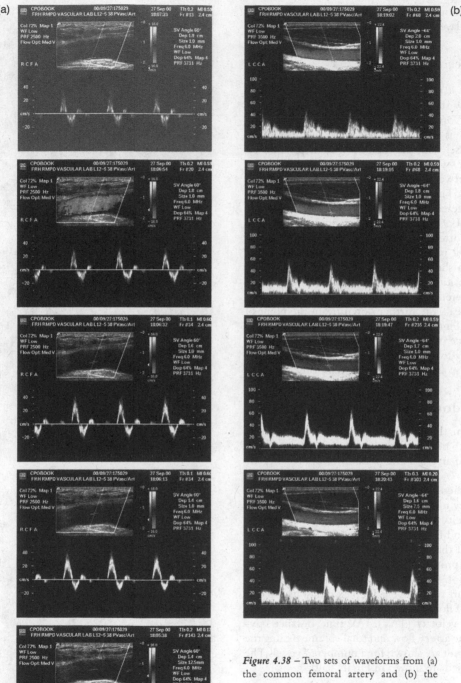

Figure 4.38 – Two sets of waveforms from (a) the common femoral artery and (b) the common carotid artery. Using a very narrow sample volume, each set shows the waveforms obtained as the sample volume is moved from the edge of the vessel to the centre line. The bottom waveform of each set shows the waveform obtained when the sample volume straddles the whole vessel.

mixing of the boundary layer with the core layers and so the boundary layer grows thicker more quickly.

Spike turbulence

In Chapter 1 it was shown that vortices produced in turbulent flow show up on the Doppler waveform as bright spikes. Vortices are generally produced when the flow velocity is highest in systole. They then travel down the vessel with the bulk flow. Their position on the Doppler waveform clearly demonstrates the difference between the flow velocity and the pulse wave velocity. The pulse wave velocity in an artery is 5–8 m s^{-1} whereas the flow velocity at peak systole is typically 0.4–0.9 m s^{-1}. Looking at a point downstream from where vortex production is occurring, the systolic peak flow will pass by very rapidly whilst the vortex will pass by a short time later as it travels at a slower speed. The position of the vortex spike on the Doppler waveform therefore occurs at a later time, relative to the systolic peak, the further downstream the point of observation (Figure 4.39). Putting this the other way, the occurrence of spike turbulence on the descending slope of the systolic peak of a waveform is indicative of possible disease a few centimetres proximally.

How fast does blood travel?

We have seen that the pulse wave velocity is high, ranging from 5 m s^{-1} in the ascending aorta to 8 m s^{-1} in the peripheral arteries. The pulse therefore reaches the extremities in < 250 ms from the commencement of systole. The actual velocity of the blood along the arteries is very much lower, typically < 1 m s^{-1} at peak systolic velocity (PSV). It is interesting to consider what the blood flow is in one cardiac cycle and what proportion of that flow occurs in systole and diastole. The velocity profile of the flow varies over the cardiac cycle (Figure 4.36) and in some vessels flow is retrograde over part of the cycle. Duplex ultrasound allows an estimate of flow to be made using the calculation of time average velocity (TAV). TAV, time, distance travelled along the artery, flow and total volume passing the measuring point are shown for a number of vessels. The waveforms used are shown in Figure 4.40.

Common carotid artery (Table 4.5)

Diameter = 7.3 mm, area = 0.42 cm^2, PSV = 68 cm s^{-1}, heart rate = 70.6 bpm.

Volume flow = 476 ml min^{-1}, thus TAV/PSV = 0.40.

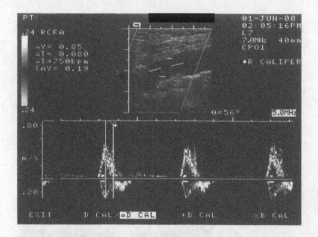

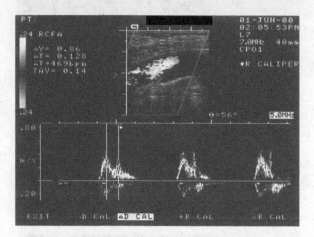

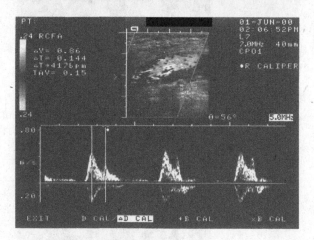

Figure 4.39 – Doppler waveforms showing spike turbulence distal to mild disease in the common femoral artery. As the distance from the origin of the vortex increases, the spike arrives at a later time after the systolic peak (80, 128, 144 ms).

Roughly speaking, if the top of the head is 40 cm above the heart, blood moves from the heart to the head in 2.5 s or three cardiac cycles. It is perhaps surprising to note that at this resting heart rate, a larger volume of blood passes the observation point during diastole than during systole.

Common femoral artery at rest (Table 4.6)

Diameter = 9.0 mm, area = 0.64 cm^2, PSV = 44 cm s^{-1}, heart rate = 65.9 bpm.

Volume flow = 117 ml min^{-1}, thus TAV/PSV = 0.36.

Assuming these figures apply to the artery from the aortic bifurcation to the foot, 100 cm say, with a mean diameter of 6 mm, then blood fills this volume of 28 ml in 14.5 s or 15 cardiac cycles. This time may be compared with the time to image the lower limb with angiography following a bolus injection of contrast into the distal aorta.

Common femoral artery following exercise (Table 4.7)

A large number of dorsiflexions of the feet whilst standing were performed to exercise the leg before making these measurements.

Diameter = 9.0 mm, area = 0.64 cm^2, PSV = 120 cm s^{-1}, heart rate = 80 bpm.

Volume flow = 1444 ml min^{-1}, thus TAV/PSV = 0.45.

Using the same figures as at rest, blood covers the distance from the aortic bifurcation to the foot in 1.2 s or 1.6 cardiac cycles. As for the carotid artery, a larger volume passes in diastole than during systole.

Posterior tibial artery at rest (Table 4.8)

Diameter = 3 mm, area = 0.071 cm^2, PSV = 44 cm s^{-1}, heart rate = 54 bpm.

Volume flow = 11.9 ml min^{-1}, TAV/PSV = 0.36.

Flow in veins

As is the case for arteries, the veins are also elastic vessels that can propagate pulsatile waveforms. Therefore, in principle, all the features such as reflection, attenuation and non-linear propagation of unsteady flow will be seen. However, in most veins the flow does not have a regular cycle such as the cardiac cycle seen in arteries.

Table 4.5 – Common cartid artery

	TAV (cm s^{-1})	Δt (ms)	Distance travelled (cm)	Flow (ml s^{-1})	Volume per cycle (ml)
Systole	27.5	280	7.56	11.34	3.18
Diastole	15.0	570	8.55	6.30	3.59
Cardiac cycle	18.9	850	16.11	7.94	6.75

Table 4.6 – Common femoral artery at rest

	TAV (cm s^{-1})	Δt (ms)	Distance travelled (cm)	Flow (ml s^{-1})	Volume per cycle (ml)
Systole	16	190	3.04	10.24	1.95
Diastole	0	720	0	0	0
Cardiac cycle	3.3	91	3.04	2.14	1.95

Table 4.7 – Common femoral artery following exercise

	TAV (cm s^{-1})	Δt (ms)	Distance travelled (cm)	Flow (ml s^{-1})	Volume per cycle (ml)
Systole	55	245	13.5	35.2	8.62
Diastole	29	505	14.7	18.6	9.39
Cardiac cycle	37.6	750	28.2	24.1	18.01

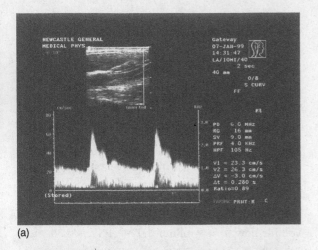

(a)

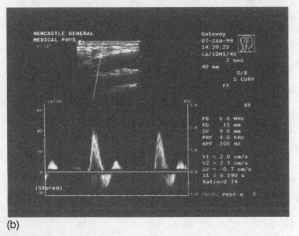

(b)

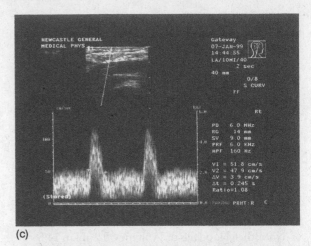

(c)

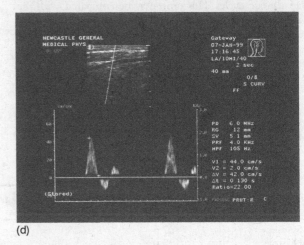

(d)

Figure 4.40 – Waveforms used in calculations to show how fast blood moves: (a) common carotid artery; (b) common femoral artery in a resting subject; (c) common femoral artery following exercise; (d) posterior tibial artery in a resting subject.

This is due to the fact that the veins are filled continuously from the low-pressure capillary bed and have valves preventing retrograde flow. An exception to this is the inferior and superior vena cava where the cardiac pulse generated by the right atrium of the heart produces pulse pressure waves that are transmitted along these vessels. This is more evident when there is

tricuspid valve regurgitation, or right-sided heart failure where right atrial pressures are raised.

Figure 4.41 shows the Doppler waveform obtained from the internal jugular vein in a young normal subject resting in a supine position. From the ECG waveform it can be seen that flow is strongly influenced

Table 4.8 – Posterior tibial artery at rest

	TAV (cm s^{-1})	Δt (ms)	Distance travelled (cm)	Flow (ml s^{-1})	Volume per cycle (ml)
Systole	16	195	3.12	0.22	0.04
Diastole	0	915	0	0	0
Cardiac cycle	2.8	1110	3.12	0.2	0.04

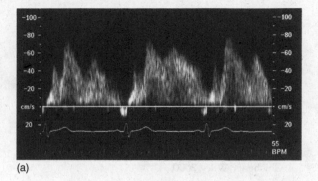

(a)

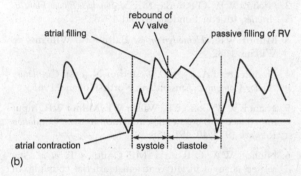

(b)

Figure 4.41 – Doppler waveform obtained from the internal jugular vein of a normal supine subject: (a) showing variation in flow with the cardiac pulse; (b) having cardiac events causing the features seen. Systole and diastole refer to the right ventricle phases.

by back pressure from the right atrium of the heart. During atrial systole flow almost ceases and with atrial contraction at the end of the passive filling phase of the ventricle there is a small 'kick back' of reverse flow. As the right atrium relaxes there is a large increase in jugular flow contributing to atrial filling. This sort of pulsatility in the jugular vein seen here in a young supine subject may be seen in an upright patient with right-sided heart failure where the right atrium is operating at raised pressure.

The vena cava has a Wormersley parameter $\alpha = \sim 8$, so the velocity profiles seen will be fairly flat. Peak flow velocities in the IVC are ~ 0.4 m s^{-1}, which give a Re = 1000–2000. As this is lower than the critical value, turbulence will not normally be seen in veins.

Venous waveforms

There are several distinct velocity waveforms that are observed in veins. Each may be explained on the basis of their mode of origin.

PULSATILE FLOW

The existence of pulsatile waveforms in the vena cava has already been discussed. Venous waveforms may also show evidence of the cardiac cycle due to the arterial pulse being directly transmitted through a very low resistance capillary bed. In the case of an arteriovenous malformation, this flow with its pulsation may be very large and is often diagnostic of the condition. An example is given in Figure 4.42.

PHASIC FLOW

Phasic flow may be defined as periods of increased then decreased or absent flow occurring over time intervals unrelated to the heart rate. It is caused by changes in intra-abdominal pressure due to respiration and by changes in peripheral flow due to the contraction of skeletal muscles. Examples are shown in Figure 4.43. With inspiration abdominal pressure increases above venous pressure, thus restricting venous outflow from the lower limbs. Retrograde flow in the veins is prevented by valves, so flow ceases. During expiration abdominal pressure decreases and venous flow can proceed. This is part of the respiratory pump mechanism that has an important function in regulating flow returning to the heart and is discussed in detail in Chapter 6.

Upon contraction of skeletal muscle, venous blood, pooling in the relaxed muscle, is driven out of the muscle towards the heart. This too has important

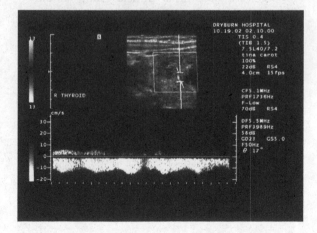

Figure 4.42 – Doppler waveform obtained from a vein in a thyroid gland with a very vascular nodule. The cardiac pulse is transmitted through the low-resistance vascular bed to the venous side.

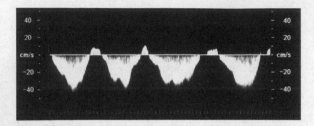

Figure 4.43 – Doppler waveform from the common femoral vein showing phasic flow with respiration.

consequences for returning blood to the heart and is the basis of the calf muscle pump, which is also discussed in Chapter 6.

Clinical note
Assessment of veins by manual compression

Normal venous flow in a subject at rest is often very low. Diagnosis of venous incompetence and occlusion is aided by manual compression of skeletal muscle. A Doppler waveform from the vein of interest is obtained whilst simultaneously compressing a group of muscles with the other hand. The rules to remember are:

- Compression of a distal muscle group should lead to a rapid enhancement of flow towards the heart – otherwise an occlusion or partial occlusion is possibly present.

- Release of a distal muscle group should produce no retrograde flow – otherwise the valves are incompetent.

- Compression of a proximal muscle group should produce no retrograde flow – otherwise the valves are incompetent.

In the iliac and common femoral veins, a similar effect to proximal compression is produced by asking the patient to perform a Valsalva manoeuvre of forced expiration against a closed glottis.

CONTINUOUS FLOW

In the smaller peripheral veins low-velocity continuous flow is seen as blood steadily moves into the veins from the capillary bed.

References

1. Evens DH, McDicken WN. *Doppler Ultrasound: Physics, Instrumentation and Clinical Applications*, 2nd edn. Chichester: Wiley, 2000.

2. Nichols WW, O'Rourke MF. *Mcdonald's Blood Flow in Arteries*, 4th edn. London: Arnold, 1998.

3. Milnor WR. *Hemodynamics*. Baltimore: Williams & Wilkins, 1982.

4. Noordergraaf A, Jager G, Westerhof N (eds). *Circulatory Analog Computers*. Amsterdam: North-Holland, 1963.

5. Nichols WW, Conti CR, Walker WE, Milnor WR. Input impedance of the systemic circulation in man. *Circulation Research* 1977; **40**: 451–458.

6. Nichols WW, O'Rourke MF, Contri CR *et al*. Age related changes in left ventricular–arterial coupling. In FCP Yin (ed.) *Vascular/Ventricular Coupling*. New York: Springer, 1987: 79–114.

7. Caro CG, Pedley TJ, Schroter RC, Seed WA. *The Mechanics of the Circulation*. Oxford: Oxford University Press, 1978.

8. Histand MB, Anliker M (1973) Circulation Research **32**: 524–529 Influence of flow and pressure on wave propagation in the canine aorta.

9. Mills CJ, Gabe IT, Gault JH *et al*. Pressure–flow relationships and vascular impedance in man. *Cardiovascular Research* 1972; **4**: 405–407.

10. Bude RO, Rubin JM, Platt JF *et al* (1994) Radiology **190** 779–784 Pulsus tardus: its cause and potential limitations in detection of arterial scenosis.

11. Pedley TJ. *The Fluid Mechanics of Large Blood Vessels*. Cambridge: Cambridge University Press, 1980.

Further reading

McDonald DA, Gessner U. Wave attenuation in visco-elastic arteries. In AL Copley (ed.) *Hemorheology*. Oxford: Pergamon, 1968: 113–125.

5

THE CARDIOVASCULAR SYSTEM – THE HEART

THE CARDIOVASCULAR SYSTEM – THE HEART

Outline

The normal function of the heart is described using ventricular pressure–volume diagrams including the cardiac cycle, myocardial contractility, heart rate and the significance of adequate venous return. Cardiac efficiency in relation to its work of supplying the circulation is discussed. Mechanisms of heart failure are described, as is the supply of oxygen via the coronary arteries.

The function of the cardiovascular system is to transport blood to all parts of the body to fulfil the physiological functions shown in Table 5.1.

It consists of the heart and the circulation. The heart is a double pump, the right and left heart, which has a pulsatile rather than a continuous action. The left and right heart supply two separate circuits connected in series, each of which arises from the heart and returns

Table 5.1 – Functions of blood and the cardiovascular system

To carry oxygen and nutrients to tissue
To carry carbon dioxide and waste products from tissue
To provide fluid to tissue
To convey secretions of ductless glands – hormones
To regulate body temperature
To protect the body from disease
To protect itself by the clotting of blood

to it (Figure 5.1). These are the pulmonary circulation, which runs from the right ventricle through the lungs to the left atrium of the heart, and the systemic circulation, which runs from the left ventricle to supply all parts of the body to return to the right atrium of the heart. With this arrangement, virtually all of the blood passes through the lungs, where oxygen and carbon dioxide are exchanged, before moving round the systemic circulation to perfuse the whole body.

Each side of the heart has two chambers, an **atrium** and a **ventricle**. The atrium receives returning blood and propels it into the ventricle. The ventricle then contracts to propel the blood round the circulation. The two pumps work in synchrony so that blood moves from the atria into the ventricles in one phase – **diastole** – and leaves the ventricles to move round the pulmonary and systemic circuits in the next phase – **systole**. The heart therefore provides the mechanical energy needed to drive blood round these two circuits. This is achieved by increasing the blood pressure on the output side, so producing a mean pressure gradient round each circuit down which blood flows. This is analogous to current flow in an electric circuit across a change in voltage. The lowest mean pressure occurs at the end of the larger systemic circuit, the right atrium. Right atrial pressure is therefore used as the pressure datum level and is taken to be 0 mmHg. A pulsatile pressure variation is superimposed on the mean pressure gradient as seen in the arteries. Since the systemic circulation is much larger than the pulmonary circulation, the left ventricle driving it is more powerful than the right ventricle producing a peak pressure of 120 mmHg compared with 25 mmHg in the right ventricle.

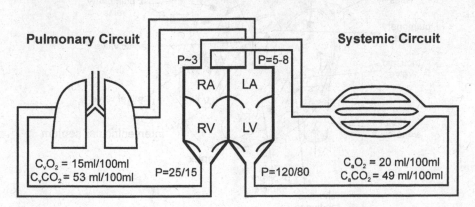

Figure 5.1 – Cardiovascular system showing right and left atria and ventricles of the heart (RA, LA, RV, LV), the pressures around the heart (systolic/diastolic), and the venous and arterial content of oxygen and carbon dioxide in blood entering and leaving the lungs in a resting subject.

Forward flow through the pulmonary and systemic circulations results from contraction of the heart muscle or **myocardium** on the four heart chambers, with **valves** preventing reverse flow (Figure 5.2). There is no active control of the valves, they are passive structures that respond to differences in pressure across them. The contracting phase of the heart chambers is known as **systole**, and the relaxation phase as **diastole**. Note that when used on their own, the terms 'systole' and 'diastole' refer to the ventricles, and to the left ventricle in particular.

Cardiac cycle

Figure 5.3 shows the relative changes in pressure and flow for the left side of heart during the cardiac cycle. During ventricular contraction the atria relax and blood flows into them from the great veins which are at a higher pressure than they are (typically 5–8 mmHg). As the ventricles relax their pressure falls below that in the atria. When ventricular pressure falls to ~5 mmHg the **arteriovenous (A-V) valves (mitral and tricuspid)** open. Blood rushes into the ventricles and up to 80% of ventricular filling occurs before atrial contraction commences. The rate of passive filling depends on the pressure difference between the great veins and the ventricles. This difference is fairly constant, so the degree of filling depends on the duration of diastole. When diastole is shortened as heart rate increases, this passive filling of the ventricles is less complete. However, at higher heart rates the shortened filling time is compensated for by a more rapid filling due to a **suction pump effect**. During ventricular contraction, the plane of the A-V valves is pulled down towards the apex of the heart facilitating filling of the atria from the veins. When the ventricles relax the valve plane springs back aiding filling of the ventricles. At this point the ventricles may even be at a negative pressure thereby sucking blood in from the atria. Following the passive-filling phase, the atria then contract increasing the pressure on the blood in the atria and forcing it into the ventricles. This active filling contributes ~20% of the ventricular filling volume. The two filling phases of the right ventricle are seen in the mitral valve waveform shown in Figure 3.10. Some blood is also regurgitated back into the great veins as there are no valves to prevent it, but the amount is limited by narrowing of the orifices as the atrial muscle round them contracts. Figure 4.41 shows this back flow in the jugular vein. At the end of filling, the ventricles contain ~120 ml blood.

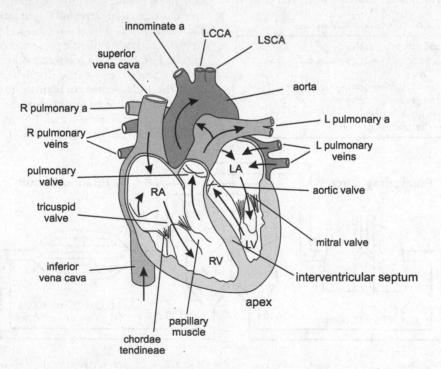

Figure 5.2 – The heart with the main anatomical features and the path of flow.

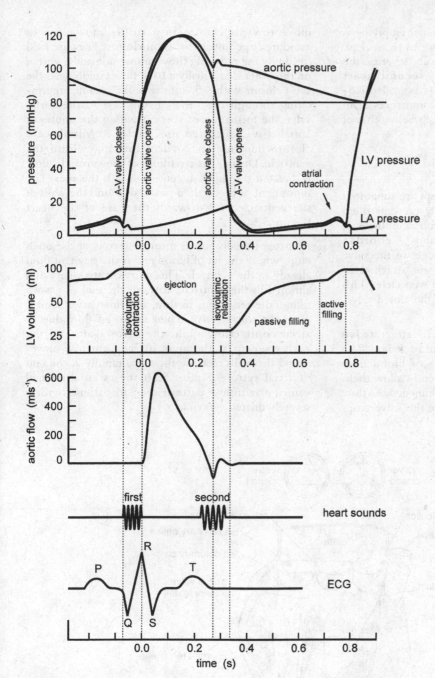

Figure 5.3 – Values and relative timings of pressure, volume and flow in the left heart over the cardiac cycle. The occurrence of heart sounds and the electrocardiogram are shown for comparison.

It is then the turn of the ventricles to contract and as soon as the ventricular pressure exceeds that in the atrium, the A-V valves close to produce the **first heart sound** as heard through a stethoscope. The ventricular pressure continues to increase on the enclosed volume of blood until the pressure exceeds that in the aorta and pulmonary artery. A phase known as **isovolumic contraction** as both inflow and outflow valves remain closed. During this phase ventricular pressure rises very rapidly. When it exceeds arterial pressure the **outflow valves (pulmonary and aortic)** open and ventricular contraction continues expelling the blood into the arteries. Valve opening occurs at 80 mmHg for the left ventricle and

15 mmHg for the right ventricle. Initial emptying is rapid but slows as the contraction begins to weaken. When the direction of flow eventually reverses, the outflow valves close producing the **second heart sound**. The ventricles then relax, a phase called **isovolumic relaxation**, and the cycle commences again when the pressure in the ventricle falls below that of the atria and the A–V valves open.

Heart valve function

The aortic and pulmonary valve cusps are supported within a fibrous ring that effectively prevents them from prolapsing into the ventricle. Prolapse of the A–V valves is prevented by fibrous strands – **chordae tendineae** – attached to the free edges of the valve cusps (Figure 5.4). They in turn are attached to **papillary muscles** deep in the ventricle. This arrangement ensures the stability of the closed valves during ventricular contraction.

Three components are required to effect **valve closure**: unsteady flow, a vortex and back flow. The valves are held open by the force of blood flow through them. **Sinuses** behind the cusps allow them to open fully so blood flow is not impeded. As flow decreases towards the end of systole the valve cusps

move towards closure in a steady movement so avoiding large impact loads on closure. They are held steady by the reducing flow on one side and a vortex on the other side. Finally a back flow rapidly seals the valve closure with < 5% of the stroke volume regurgitating through the valve. In the case of the aortic valve, the formation of vortices within the sinuses of Valsalva was discussed in Chapter 3. Mitral valve closure depends on vortices forming within the ventricle. During passive filling of the ventricle, flow is directed through the centre towards the apex. The movement of blood then proceeds round the walls of the ventricle back towards the base of the heart (Figure 5.5a).

A vortex initially forms round the rims of the open cusps where the jet of blood enters the stagnant fluid already in the ventricle. This vortex is stationary and almost fills the ventricle. Towards the end of passive filling, the reduction in flow and this vortex almost close the mitral valve. Then increased flow due to atrial contraction opens the valve again and the vortex set up at the apex of the ventricle moves round the walls to close the valve rapidly at the end of atrial systole. Figure 5.5b shows an abnormal ventricular inflow pattern seen in patients with a severely dilated ventricle.

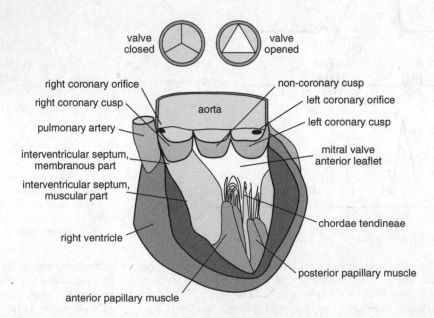

Figure 5.4 – Left ventricle with the aortic valve opened up to show the semilunar cusps and orifices of the coronary arteries behind the cusps. To the left side of the ventricle the papillary muscles and chordae tendineae support the leaflet of the mitral valve. The open and closed position of the aortic valve leaflets is indicated.

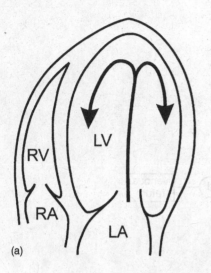 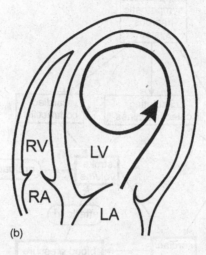

(a)　(b)

Figure 5.5 – Inflow patterns into the left ventricle with (a) normal inflow where early diastolic flow is directed towards the apex and later flow is forced round the walls back towards the base, and (b) inflow into a dilated ventricle where flow is directed towards the lateral wall forming a rotating pattern.[1]

Clinical note
Left ventricular flow patterns on colour Doppler examination

Normal and abnormal ventricular flow patterns such as those shown in Figure 5.5 may be detected on colour Doppler examination. Two distinct abnormal patterns may be recognised. In the first type, flow towards the apex is seen along the lateral wall and continues throughout both phases of ventricular filling. Simultaneously flow towards the base of the heart is seen along the interventricular septum. That is the pattern seen in Figure 5.5b. It is seen in patients with a severely dilated ventricle, increasing the angle between the anterior mitral valve leaflet and the intraventricular septum.

The second type has a delay of 160–300 ms between the maximum velocity measured near the apex and the maximum velocity in the mitral valve orifice. The velocities near the apex are also higher than in normal subjects. This is due to a circular ring vertex, similar to that seen in a smoke ring, moving from the valve towards the apex. The effect may be seen on colour-flow imaging. This type of flow is seen in patients with a dilated ventricle and a low ejection fraction.

Cardiac output

Table 5.2 shows the typical cardiac output at rest for a supine subject.

Cardiac output (CO) is the volume flow from the heart. Since the heart is a pulsatile pump, it is the product of the **heart rate** (HR) and the volume discharged per beat, known as the **stroke volume** (SV):

$$CO = HR \times SV$$

Cardiac Output Equation

The factors controlling cardiac output are summarised in Figure 5.6.

Circulation as a supplier of oxygen

As indicated above, one of the main purposes of the circulation is to carry oxygen (O_2) to all tissues in the body. The failure of the circulation to perfuse any vascular bed with O_2 will lead very rapidly to a critical situation

Table 5.2 – Typical cardiac output at rest for a supine subject

Heart rate (bpm)	70
Cardiac output (l min^{-1})	5.6
LV end-diastolic volume (ml)	145
LV end-systolic volume (ml)	65
Stroke volume (ml)	80
Ejection fraction	0.55

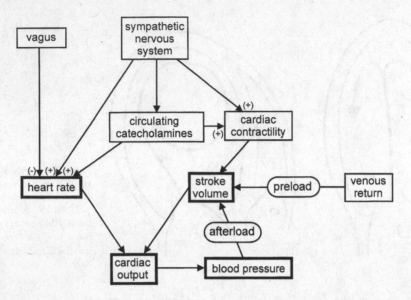

Figure 5.6 – Factors controlling cardiac output.

for the tissue supplied by that route as it becomes ischaemic. As blood passes through the lung it typically enters the pulmonary circulation 75% full of O_2 and leaves it 98–100% full. The difference of ~25% between venous and arterial blood is known as the **oxygen extraction ratio (OER)**. The absolute amount of O_2 carried in the blood depends on the haematocrit, OER, the partial pressure of O_2 in inspired air and O_2 uptake in the lung. With a lung diffusion surface area of 70–100 m² for a pulmonary capillary volume of 100 ml, O_2 uptake is not normally a problem. Reduced O_2 uptake can arise when there is lung disease or **pulmonary shunting**. This occurs if blood passes through the lung too quickly to complete gas exchange or gas exchange is otherwise impeded so blood leaves the lung from these parts with O_2 pressure close to venous levels. Blood draining into the thebsian veins in the heart and that passing through the bronchial and pleural circulation bypass the lung. The total amount of unoxygenated blood entering the left side of the heart normally accounts for 2–5% of cardiac output. Normal values for the O_2 and carbon dioxide (CO_2) content of blood are shown in Table 5.3.

Table 5.3 – Oxygen and carbon dioxide content and partial pressures in blood at resting levels

		(ml 100 ml⁻¹)		(mmHg)
Arterial blood	CaO_2	20	PaO_2	100
	$CaCO_2$	49	$PaCO_2$	40
Venous blood	CvO_2	15	PvO_2	40
(RA)	$CvCO_2$	53	$PvCO_2$	46

Technical note
Expressing oxygen and carbon dioxide levels

The amount of O_2 and CO_2 carried in air, blood or other tissue may be expressed as a volume or pressure. The volume of a gas changes with temperature and pressure, so a standard or normal temperature and pressure is used when making comparisons. The temperature used is 20°C and the pressure is 760 mmHg, which is the mean pressure of the atmosphere (air) at sea level.

Volume description

The volume of a gas in blood is expressed in millilitres per 100 ml (i.e. ml 100 ml⁻¹) blood. This is the volume the gas would occupy in its gaseous form at normal temperature and pressure; for example, arterial O_2 content CaO_2 = 20 ml 100 ml⁻¹. For a tissue, O_2 content may be expressed as millilitres per 100 g (i.e. ml 100 g⁻¹) tissue.

Pressure description

The pressure of a given volume of a mixture of gases, such as air, can be considered to be made up of the sum of the pressures of each constituent gas, assuming they alone occupied the same volume at the same temperature. This is Dalton's law of **partial pressures**. For example, 21% of air is O_2, so that in dry air at normal temperature and pressure, the partial pressure of $O_2 = 0.21 \times 760 = 160$ mmHg, and the partial pressure of CO_2 is $0.033 \times 760 = 25$ mmHg. Within the alveoli of the lung the inhaled air is saturated with water vapour at 36°C. This water vapour also contributes to the total air pressure, and the partial pressure of O_2 in the alveoli is reduced to 100 mmHg.

The O_2 content of any tissue can be expressed as a partial pressure that may be compared with the partial pressure in the blood perfusing it. Where two regions with different partial pressures are adjacent, O_2 molecules will tend to move out of the high-pressure region to the low-pressure one by a process of diffusion similar to that of osmosis for solutes in liquids. This will continue until the partial pressures reach equilibrium. This process is seen in gas transfer across the alveolar epithelium in the lung.

Fick principle

The **Fick principle** relates the total O_2 uptake of the body $\dot{V}O_2$ (l min^{-1}) to the difference in O_2 content of the arterial blood leaving the heart and venous blood returning to the right atrium AVO_2 *diff* (ml 100 ml^{-1} blood).

$$\dot{V}O_2 = HR \times SV \times AVO_2 \; diff$$

It demonstrates that in order for the supply of O_2 to tissue to be maintained or increased, the cardiac output must increase through a higher heart rate HR or increased stroke volume, or that tissue must extract a greater proportion of O_2 carried by the blood. Oxygen uptake will be at its maximum limit when heart rate, stroke volume and O_2 extraction are all at their maximum levels. This is known as $\dot{V}O_2$ *max*, and will be reached when a large percentage of the skeletal muscle mass is maximally exercised. The difference between resting $\dot{V}O_2$ and $\dot{V}O_2$ *max* is a measure of the reserve capacity for exercise, or how near the resting body is to its O_2 limit. This is shown for three examples in Figure 5.7, a normally active subject, an endurance athlete and a

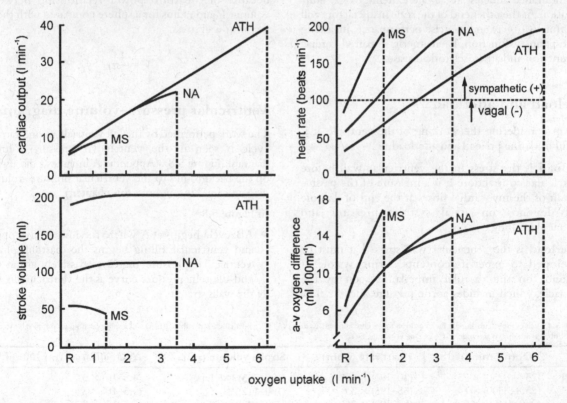

Figure 5.7 – Four determinants of $\dot{V}O_2$ *max* for a subject with pure mitral valve stenosis (MS), a normally active subject (NA) and an élite endurance athlete (ATH). Broken vertical lines show VO_2 *max* in each case.[2]

patient with pure mitral valve stenosis (Table 5.4). Pure mitral valve stenosis with no cardiac failure, pulmonary hypertension or congestion and with approximately normal cardiac output at rest is used as a model for low maximal cardiac output.[2]

Notes:

- In all of these cases the maximum AVO_2 *diff* is similar but the mitral stenosis patient is operating at a slightly elevated level of O_2 extraction even at rest.

- Stroke volume can change the least but its absolute value varies significantly between the three cases. In the mitral stenosis patient ventricular filling is greatly restricted by the stenosed valve and stroke volume actually decreases at higher heart rates because of reduced filling time. In the athlete, stroke volume is increased through sustained training giving both increased filling and contractility.

- Maximum heart rate in each case is ~195 bpm. The difference in range between the three cases is in the resting heart rate.

- Endurance athletes are at one extreme of O_2 utilisation. At the other end of the scale many factors will limit $\dot{V}O_2$ *max* and exercise performance, including respiratory function, haematocrit, impaired cardiac function and atherosclerotic disease.

Preload and afterload

When considering the working of the ventricle, it is useful to define preload and afterload.

Preload is the stress in the ventricular wall before ventricular contraction. It is a measure of the passive stretch of the myocardial fibres at the end of diastole and depends on atrial systolic pressure and ventricular filling.

Afterload is the ventricular wall stress that must be developed to expel its contents during systole. It depends on the vascular impedance seen by the ventricle, which includes aortic pressure and the flow resistance of the aortic valve. The presence of aortic valve stenosis increases resistance in the outflow tract. The ventricular wall must then expend more energy and develop a greater force to overcome the resistance.

Ascending aortic pressure has been used as a measure of afterload when considering the working efficiency of the heart. However, this is an approximation as wall stress depends on ventricular pressure P, ventricular radius r and wall thickness h, and these vary throughout ventricular ejection.

For a pseudo-spherical volume such as the ventricle, wall stress σ (Chapter 3) is given by:

$$\sigma = \frac{P\pi r^2}{h}$$

As ejection occurs, the pressure in the ventricle increases but the volume decreases. In a normal heart, wall tension falls during ventricular ejection as the radius decreases more rapidly than the ventricular pressure increases to expel the blood. This occurs because of the third power relationship between volume V and radius for a sphere compared with the r^2 factor in wall stress:

$$V = \frac{4}{3}\pi r^3$$

Ventricular pressure–volume diagram

The work performed by the left ventricle in one cardiac cycle is seen in the ventricular pressure–volume diagram (Figure 5.8). (Appendix A includes a discussion on the background to the ventricular pressure–volume diagrams used throughout this chapter.)

In Figure 5.8:

- AB: cycle begins at A where the mitral valve opens and ventricular filling begins the diastolic phase. Ventricular pressure increases passively along the end–diastolic pressure curve as the ventricle fills and the walls stretch.

Table 5.4 –Values for calculating the Fick equation for an élite endurance athlete (ATH), a normally active subject (NA) and a subject with pure mitral valve stenosis (MS). Subjects are shown as (range, rest – $\dot{V}O_2$ *max*) × range factor

	$\dot{V}O_2$ (ml min^{-1})	=	Heart rate (bpm)	×	Stroke volume (ml)	×	AVO$_2$ *difference* (ml 100 ml^{-1})
ATH	(250–6,250) × 25		(30–190) × 6.4		(190–205) × 1.1		(4.5–16) × 3.7
NA	(250–3,500) × 14		(55–195) × 3.6		(100–112) × 1.1		(4.5–16) × 3.7
MS	(250–1,400) × 5.6		(83–190) × 2.3		(53–43) × 0.8		(5.5–17) × 3.1

Rowell (1993).[2]

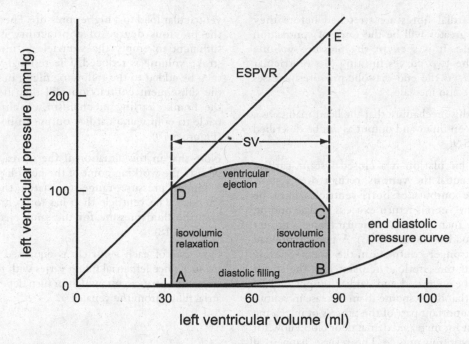

Figure 5.8 – Left ventricular pressure–volume diagram of the normal left ventricle with the subject at rest. ESPVR, end-systolic pressure–volume relation.

- BC: mitral valve closes and ventricular contraction begins the systolic phase. Ventricular pressure increases rapidly against a fixed volume of blood, the isovolumic contraction phase.

- CD: aortic valve opens and ejection begins. In the normal heart ventricular pressure increases and then decreases as ventricular relaxation commences.

- DA: ejection ends when ventricular pressure equals a point on the end-systolic pressure–volume relation curve. The aortic valve closes. Isovolumic relaxation occurs and the cycle is complete.

Notes:

- The **end-systolic pressure–volume relation (ESPVR)** is the curve that would be obtained if the ventricle contracted to peak systolic pressure with no ejection of blood taking place, for example BE or AD.

- **Stroke volume** (SV) is the difference between the end-diastolic volume ED_{vol} (BC) and the end-systolic volume (AD).

- **Ejection fraction** (EF) is the fractional emptying of the ventricle:

$$EF = \frac{SV}{ED_{vol}}$$

EF is normally 0.55 at rest, rising to 0.75 at maximum output. EF < 0.5 at rest or a failure to increase with exercise or with autonomic stimulation is a sign of significant LV impairment.

- Preload is the wall stress at B; afterload is the wall stress over ventricular ejection CD.

- The ventricle works both in increasing the fluid pressure and in ejecting its volume of blood into the aorta. The energy imparted to the ejected blood by the ventricle in one cycle is therefore equal to the shaded area inside the pressure–volume curve, i.e. change in pressure × change in volume (recall: work = force × distance moved). This is known as the **external work** of the heart.

Myocardial contractility

Stroke volume depends on ventricular filling, the contractility of myocardium during ventricular systole which determines the degree of emptying, and ventricular afterload.

The force of ventricular contraction increases with increasing preload or end-diastolic volume. This is known as the **Frank–Starling mechanism** and results from the fact that the greater the length to which myocardial fibres are stretched before they contract, the greater will be the force of contraction when they do. It is seen in the pressure–volume diagram as the two curves limiting the ventricular working cycle. As the end-diastolic pressure increases so the ESPVR also increases.

It is through this mechanism that the heart maintains a balance between input and output as can be described using Figure 5.9.

Because the circulation is a closed system, cardiac output must equal the **venous return** over a short time and the outputs of both ventricles must be matched. If the venous return exceeds cardiac output, atrial pressure increases, so ventricular filling is greater and the preload is increased (B). A greater preload produces a stronger contraction, the Frank–Starling mechanism. If the afterload remains low, the stroke volume will be increased and cardiac output will be higher. Note that this response to an increase in venous return is an important part of the process of increasing cardiac output for increased demand for blood flow, for example in working muscle. The reverse happens if cardiac output is higher than the venous return. Preload is reduced, contractility is reduced and stroke volume falls.

Figure 5.9 also shows the effect of increasing the afterload (C) caused, for example, by increasing peripheral vascular resistance or a previously high stroke volume. In this case more energy of the ventricular contraction must go into raising the

ventricular load to a higher pressure. The result is that the previous degree of contractility is no longer sufficient to empty the ventricle as much and the stroke volume is reduced. The residual volume will then be added to the following filling in diastole and the subsequent contraction will then be greater by the Frank–Starling mechanism, enabling the ventricle to empty and cardiac output to be maintained (Figure 5.10).

Note that in this situation if the increased afterload persists, the working point of the heart has to move to a higher pressure range to match the increased afterload. The ventricle then has to do more work to raise the fluid pressure for the same ejected volume (Figure 5.18).

Flow out of each ventricle is equalised in a similar manner since left atrial filling varies with flow through the pulmonary circuit, which in turn depends on right atrial filling from the vena cava.

Clinical note
Irregular heart beats

In patients with irregular heart rates or with ectopic beats occurring, the peak systolic velocity seen in the beat following a longer time interval will be greater than for beats occurring with shorter intervals (Figure 5.11). This is due to the action of the Frank–Starling mechanism and the increased recovery in cell calcium concentration. Filling of the ventricle will be greater in a longer time interval and subsequent systolic contraction will be greater producing a larger stroke volume in the following systole.

Unless there are three or four consecutive beats of similar duration and magnitude, it is not really possible to make meaningful velocity measurements in these patients. The assessment then has to be qualitative, looking at features in the shape of Doppler waveforms such as systolic rise time, presence of a systolic window, type of diastolic flow, etc. A qualitative indication of high or low velocities may be given together with observation of the width of the lumen on colour Doppler.

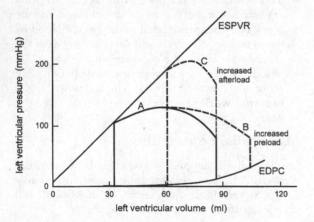

Figure 5.9 – Left ventricular pressure–volume curves for normal resting LV (A), increased preload producing an increased ejection fraction (B) and increased afterload (C) where the ejection fraction is maintained by the heart operating at a higher systolic pressure.

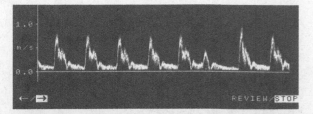

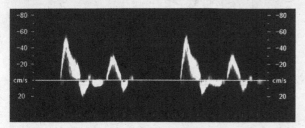

Figure 5.10 – Two examples of the Frank–Starling mechanism operating when there is an irregular heart rate. A short interval is succeeded by a reduced stroke volume, a longer interval by an increased stroke volume.

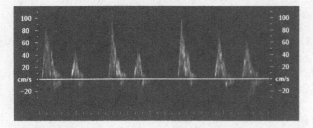

Figure 5.11 – Waveform from a patient with an irregular heart rate. Every systolic peak is a different height and a meaningful PSV measurement cannot be made.

Sympathetic activity increasing contractility

In addition to the Frank–Starling mechanism, myocardial contractility is also increased by sympathetic neural stimulation and circulating hormones that act on the myocardium. These stimuli have the effect of shifting the ESPVR curve above the unstimulated level (Figure 5.12). This increases the stroke volume by increasing the ejection fraction (B). In the case of an increased afterload it enables stroke volume to be maintained (C).

The limit of end-diastolic volume, and hence stroke volume, is set by the constraint of the **pericardium** surrounding the heart. In patients who have had their pericardium cut, stroke volume can be greater than normal. Figure 5.13 shows how stroke volume increases

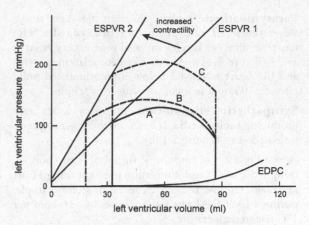

Figure 5.12 – Left ventricular pressure–volume curves with a change in myocardial contractility. An increase in contractility (ESVPR 2) enables an increase in stroke volume through an increased ejection fraction (B) or by maintenance of stroke volume with increased afterload (C).

with exercise in an upright subject. Notice how ejection fraction increases to 85% at peak exercise.

The contractility of the atria is affected by arterial blood pressure through the baroreceptor reflex described below, so that the ventricular preload and hence filling can be controlled.

Heart rate

Heart rate is under the control of circulating hormones (see Chapter 6) and both parasympathetic and sympathetic branches of the autonomic nervous system.

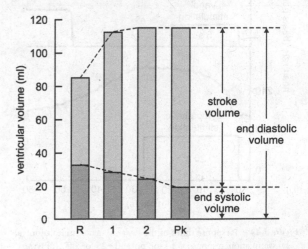

Figure 5.13 – Left ventricular volumes at rest (R), mild exercise (1), moderate exercise (2) and peak level exercise (Pk) in normal young upright subjects. At peak exercise the ejection fraction was 85%.[2]

Parasympathetic activity through the vagus nerve slows the heart rate producing **bradycardia**. The response time of changes in vagal tone is very rapid at 1–2 s (Figure 5.14a). At rest vagal stimulation is active and the heart is slowed below its unstimulated pulse rate of ~105 bpm in a young adult to ~70 bpm.

Sympathetic stimulation increases heart rate producing **tachycardia**. It has a much longer response time of 5–15 s (Figure 5.14b).

At rest both sets of autonomic stimulation are continuously active with vagal stimulation predominating. Heart rate is also sensitive to body temperature so, for example, during a fever the heart rate increases by ~10 bpm per 1°C rise in temperature.

When there is a demand for increased cardiac output during exercise, most of the increase in heart rate up to 100 bpm results from withdrawal of vagal tone (Figure 5.15). An increase > 100 bpm is a result of sympathetic stimulation. Since vagal tone can be withdrawn very rapidly, the response to immediate demand depends on the difference between resting heart rate and 100 bpm. Figure 5.7 shows that the athlete can achieve an increase in cardiac output of 14 l min⁻¹ or 35% of his maximal cardiac output through vagal withdrawal

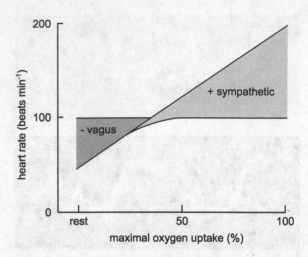

Figure 5.15 – Relative contribution of sympathetic and parasympathetic nervous systems to the rise in heart rate during exercise.[2]

alone. For the patient with mitral valve stenosis, vagal withdrawal only increases cardiac output by 0.85 l min⁻¹. Any further increase in heart rate occurs more slowly as sympathetic stimulation increases. In all subjects the maximum heart rate is 180–200 bpm.

Diastolic period

As heart rate increases, the decrease in the length of diastole is greater than that of systole. This means that ventricular filling time is reduced as heart rate increases from 660 ms at 60 bpm to 130 ms at 180 bpm (Figure 5.16).

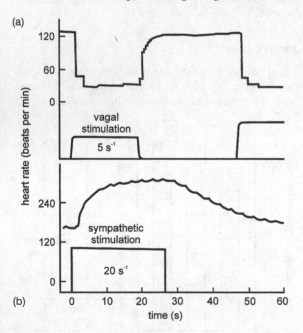

Figure 5.14 – Response times of the heart to neural stimulation: (a) vagal stimulation: response < 1 s for 'on' and ~2 s for 'off'; (b) sympathetic stimulation: response time is much slower. The on response was not fully complete for 10–20 s. The off response was even slower (adapted from Warner and Cox 1962).[2,3]

> ### Clinical note
> #### *Doppler waveform measurements within a cardiac cycle*
>
> Care needs to be taken when defining and using measurements on Doppler waveforms that depend on the timing within the cardiac cycle. The length of systole changes very little with heart rate (Figure 5.16). A measurement such as systolic rise time is therefore relatively constant over a wide range of heart rate. On the other hand, the length of diastole shows a large variation with heart rate. End-diastolic velocity may therefore vary significantly with heart rate as the maximum velocity tends to fall throughout diastole. It is more reliable to measure diastolic velocity at a fixed time interval after the start of systole (Figure 5.17).

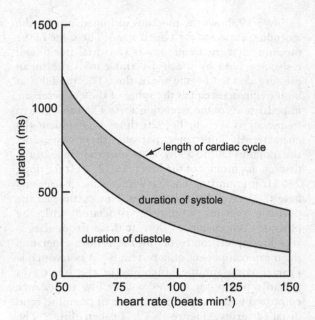

Figure 5.16 – Reduction in the duration of diastole as heart rate increases.[4]

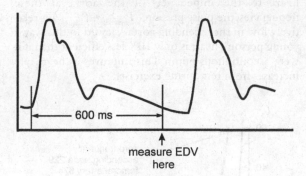

Figure 5.17 – There is a need for caution when making measurements that depend on the length of the cardiac cycle, e.g. end-diastolic velocity (EDV).

Cardiac output versus heart rate

Over the range 60–90 bpm the shorter filling time means that stroke volume reduces as heart rate increases so that cardiac output (CO = SV × HR) is maintained at a constant level, assuming venous return stays constant. Above 100 bpm, in the tachycardia range, contractility also increases as a result of the sympathetic stimulation and calcium flux into and out of the myocardial cells. Therefore, although filling time is reduced, ejection fraction increases

and, with the increase in heart rate, cardiac output increases. Above 170 bpm, ventricular filling is severely impaired as the diastolic interval becomes shorter than the rapid filling phase. Below 40 bpm, filling is complete, but the reduction in heart rate reduces cardiac output.

Cardiac efficiency

The work the ventricle does on the ejected volume of blood equals the area inside the closed pressure–volume curve (Figure 5.8). This may be considered to be the useful work of the heart. However, during isovolumic contraction the myocardium must also increase the pressure of the residual volume of blood in addition to the ejected volume. This is shown as the total shaded area in Figure 5.18a. The O_2 consumption of the heart, which is a good measure of the work it does, is proportional to this larger area.

A low ejection fraction giving a large residual volume, or a high afterload requiring elevated ventricular pressure to eject the blood, is therefore very expensive in terms of the work the heart has to do to maintain cardiac output. Figure 5.18b shows that increasing stroke volume by increasing ventricular filling requires a lower excess expenditure of energy than maintaining stroke volume but with an increased afterload.

Viewed simply as a mechanical device, cardiac efficiency may be defined as the ratio of the useful work produced to the total energy expended. The useful work in this case is volume output into a circulation at an elevated pressure. Calculating the useful work to the total energy expended by measuring O_2 consumption, the efficiency of the left ventricle has been estimated to average ~23%.

Heart-circulation input impedance

So far we have considered ventricular afterload as the systolic wall stress in the ventricle, which may be approximated by the aortic pressure into which the ventricle must eject its volume of blood. This is a useful approach when considering the function of the heart itself. However, when looking at the relationship of the heart as a pulsatile pump to the rest of the circulation, the hydraulic load seen by the heart is the vascular impedance of the ascending aorta. This forms the input impedance of the circulation as seen by the

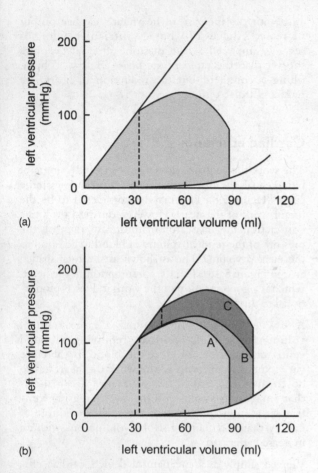

(a)

(b)

Figure 5.18 – Left ventricular pressure–volume diagrams: (a) total work that must be done by the heart (shaded area); (b) extra work required to increase stroke volume (B) and maintain stroke volume against increased afterload (C), compared with normal heart (A).

heart (see Chapter 4) and is completely independent of the properties or function of the heart itself. It determines what pressure and flow wave is generated by a given ventricular ejection wave and depends on three components: resistance to flow, vessel compliance and reflections from distal sites. This gives another route to considering the efficiency of the heart as a pump. Generally speaking a continuous pump would be more efficient than a pulsatile pump in producing a continuous flow to distal tissues. Accelerating and decelerating blood is wasteful of energy in achieving this. From this point of view, the zero-frequency mean flow component of blood flow is the useful part and the oscillatory components are wasteful of energy.

Figure 5.19 shows the modulus of impedance for the ascending aorta and for a distal artery. The value of the modulus at zero frequency is the total peripheral resistance seen by the heart and equals the mean pressure divided by the mean flow. The modulus at high frequencies equals the value of the characteristic impedance Z_0 of the ascending aorta. The value at zero frequency is seen to be ~20 times higher than the characteristic impedance. Between these two values the modulus falls to a low value over the range of the first few harmonics of the heart rate (2–8 Hz for dogs; 2–6 Hz for humans). These low impedance harmonics have the largest flow amplitudes. This means that the pulsatile pressure amplitude associated with the pulsatile components of flow at these frequencies is very low in relation to the mean pressure generating the mean component of flow. This is a very favourable characteristic for the efficiency of the heart as a pulsatile pump, for it 'sees' a very low impedance compared with the high impedance of the more rigid distal arteries (Figure 5.19, broken line). The peripheral vascular resistance is the dominant value, which would also be the case were the heart a continuous pump. As a result of this matching of the heart to the impedance of the aorta at these frequencies, the pulse pressure ($P_{\text{systolic}} - P_{\text{diastolic}}$) is relatively low in the ascending aorta. Viewed in this way, a young person's heart is only 10% less efficient than if it were a continuous pump. This improves as heart rate increases from rest during exercise.

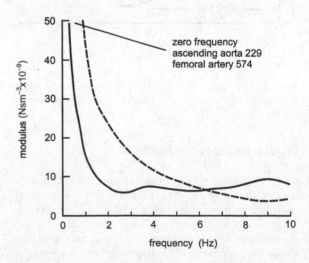

Figure 5.19 – Impedance modulus for the ascending aorta (solid line) and femoral artery (broken line) in a canine model (adapted from O'Rourke 1967).[5]

There are four main factors contributing to this energy efficient low-input impedance:

- The high distensibility of the proximal aorta gives it the lowest characteristic impedance of any systemic artery. The left ventricle 'sees' this low characteristic impedance rather than the higher characteristic impedance of the more distal arteries.

- Peripheral wave reflection produces a dip in impedance modulus at low frequencies thereby reducing the value of the already low characteristic impedance of the aorta still further.

- The relationship between body length and heart rate is such that the peripheral reflections arrive in a time interval that produces the low impedance at the right frequency. In other words, there is a tuning effect between heart rate and body length.

- The asymmetry of the heart's location increases the range of favourable pulse frequencies. The heart is closer to upper limb reflection sites than to lower limb ones, which extends the period over which reflections arrive. This is also affected by the dispersion of reflecting sites across the peripheral vasculature which broadens the range of frequencies over which impedance is low. The extended range of frequencies with low impedance this produces ensures that the impedance remains favourable over the physiological range of heart rate.

The benefit of this low-input impedance 'seen' by the heart is greatest in early adulthood and is gradually lost with age. It has been shown that a heart rate that is ideal for the systemic circulation is also well suited to the pulmonary circulation.

Heart failure

Heart failure is a fall in cardiac output to a level insufficient to meet the metabolic demands of the body, or it can only do so if the cardiac filling pressures are abnormally high, or both. These are known respectively as forward failure and backward failure.[6] It can result from a wide range of factors that affect cardiac function in three ways: impaired contractility, increased afterload and impaired ventricular filling. Impairment due to contractility or afterload is known as **systolic dysfunction** and that due to ventricular filling or preload as **diastolic dysfunction**.

Left-sided heart failure

SYSTOLIC DYSFUNCTION

Systolic dysfunction arises in the following ways:

- **Reduced contractility** due to myocardial fibrosis or impaired myocyte function and results in a lower ESPVR curve (Figure 5.20). The ejection fraction is then reduced, which leads to increased residual volume and an increased preload which the Frank–Starling mechanism partially compensates for by increasing stroke volume.

- **Increase in afterload**, e.g. chronic hypertension or aortic valve stenosis. Energy is then expended in raising the ventricular pressure to a higher level with less contraction of the myocardium during ejection resulting in a smaller stroke volume.

- **Dilated ventricle**: from the definition of afterload, as the stress σ develops in the ventricular wall during systole, we can see that afterload in a dilated ventricle is increased since the radius r of the ventricle is increased:

$$\sigma = \frac{P\pi r^2}{h}$$

The myocardium responds to chronic loading by increasing its thickness h, becoming hypertrophied. This reduces the wall stress but results in a less compliant wall. In the case of pressure overload (high afterload), it results in wall thickening without

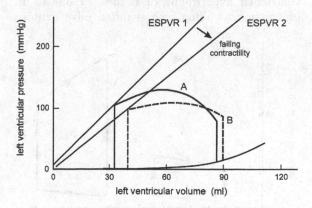

Figure 5.20 – Left ventricular pressure–volume for a heart with systolic dysfunction. 'A' is a normal pressure–volume curve. Reduced contractility moves ESPVR from 1 to 2 reducing end-systolic volume (B). This is partially compensated for by increased end-diastolic volume and the Frank–Starling mechanism.

an increase in ventricular volume, known as **concentric hypertrophy**. In the case of volume overload (high preload), there is an increase in wall thickness and chamber radius, known as **eccentric hypertrophy**. When a heart becomes dilated the ventricle can no longer collapse as much during ejection and wall tension must then continue to increase throughout the ejection phase in order to expel the blood (Figure 5.21).

During diastole the persistently elevated left ventricular pressure is transmitted in a retrograde direction through the open mitral valve to the left atrium, and then to the pulmonary veins and capillaries. A pulmonary capillary transmural pressure >20 mmHg will result in **pulmonary oedema** and congestion. This causes breathlessness or **dyspnoea** on exertion, which is a prominent symptom of left ventricular failure. Breathlessness upon lying supine also occurs. This is because the heart cannot pump the increased venous return that occurs when blood from the dependent parts is redistributed to the thorax on lying down. Figure 5.22 shows the effect of wave reflection in the aorta with age and heart failure. The reflected wave in the aorta still occurs in heart failure because the impedance does not change. However, instead of adding to pressure it subtracts from flow because the heart cannot sustain the raised pressure and the aortic valve closes restricting flow.

DIASTOLIC DYSFUNCTION

Diastolic dysfunction may be due to impaired ventricular relaxation and filling, for example due to ventricular hypertrophy or fibrosis, or due to an obstruction to filling such as mitral valve stenosis.

Ventricular compliance during filling is the ratio of the change in volume for a given change in pressure:

$$\text{Compliance} = \frac{\Delta \text{ volume}}{\Delta \text{ pressure}}$$

If the compliance is reduced with an increase in wall stiffness, the pressure will increase more rapidly than normal as the ventricle fills. This results in the end-diastolic volume curve becoming steeper and preload is lower resulting in a decreased stroke volume (Figure 5.23).

As in systolic dysfunction, the elevated diastolic pressures are transmitted in a retrograde direction to the pulmonary circulation and systemic veins.

Right-sided heart failure

The right ventricle is a thin-walled and highly compliant chamber that accepts blood at very low pressure and ejects it against a low pulmonary vascular resistance. It can therefore accept a wide range of venous filling volumes without a significant increase in its filling pressure. It is, however, susceptible to failure in the presence of increased afterload such as acute pulmonary embolism or advanced pulmonary disease. Most right ventricular failure is in fact due to left heart failure, resulting from increased pulmonary pressures due to left ventricular dysfunction. Pressures are transmitted back into the central veins causing distension and pulsation in the jugular vein, engorgement of the hepatosplenic veins and peripheral oedema. These effects form what is commonly called **congestive heart failure**. Figure 5.24 shows an example of pulsatile flow transmitted in the venous system to the popliteal vein. Note the rapid pulse of 90 bpm that is also typical of heart failure.

Compensatory mechanisms for heart failure

In addition to the Frank–Starling mechanism and vessel wall hypertrophy, neural–hormonal stimulation occurs to maintain blood pressure as cardiac output decreases in the failing heart. The mechanisms are discussed in more detail in Chapter 6 under control of blood pressure. The net effect is that peripheral resistance is increased raising arterial pressure, and total intravascular fluid volume is increased by reducing excretion of water and salt by the kidneys. This increases left ventricular preload so maximising stroke volume by the Frank–Starling mechanism.

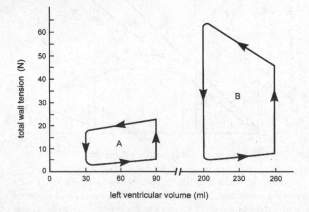

Figure 5.21 – Total wall tension–volume curves for a normal-sized heart (A) and a dilated heart (B) for one cardiac cycle.[7]

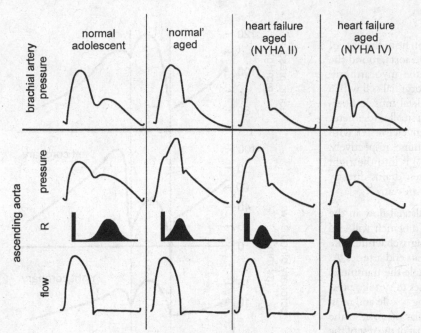

Figure 5.22 – Effects of wave reflection on brachial artery pressure and aortic pressure and flow due to ageing and the development of heart failure in a patient with isolated systolic hypertension. 'R' shows the effect of wave reflection with the effect on pressure shown above the line and flow shown below the line. Note that in the case of heart failure the effect is to reduce flow rather than to increase pressure in the ascending aorta.[8]

In the early stages of heart failure these changes are beneficial and serve to maintain blood pressure. However, chronic activation of them often proves deleterious to the failing heart. The ability of the heart to increase output to meet extra demand is then minimal and such demands may precipitate severe heart failure.

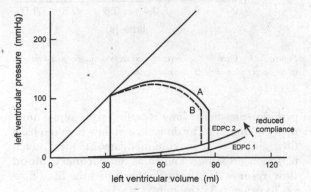

Figure 5.23 – Left ventricular pressure–volume for a heart with diastolic dysfunction. 'A' is a normal heart. Reduced ventricular compliance raises the rate of increase in end-diastolic pressure from EDPC 1 to EDPC 2. This results in reduced end-diastolic volume and reduced stroke volume (B).

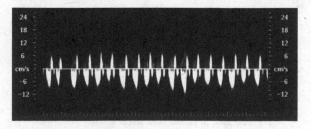

Figure 5.24 – Pulsatile Doppler waveform in the popliteal vein of a patient with cardiac failure.

Clinical note
Waveforms seen in patients with low cardiac output

In the investigation of carotid or other arteries the observation of waveforms with a normal waveform shape but low peak systolic velocity may be due to low cardiac output. If they are due to a cardiac problem then the low velocities will be seen bilaterally and throughout the arterial tree, assuming there is no local stenosis. Other causes of low peak systolic velocity that must be considered are ectactic vessels, where it may be seen from the volume flow equation that velocities will be low in a wide vessel, or the presence of distal disease causing reduced flow in the vessels. These other causes would themselves have to be bilateral to cause the effect seen. As an example, waveforms with a normal shape but PSV $\leq$ 40 cm^{-1} seen throughout the carotid arteries are likely to be due to low cardiac output.

Coronary blood flow

The right and left coronary arteries run from the base of the sinus of Valsalva, at the root of the aorta, round the epicardium sending branches into the myocardium. There they branch to supply each myocardial cell with a capillary supply. Compared with skeletal muscle fibres (diameter 50 μm), myocytes are much smaller (diameter 17 μm), and their capillary density is much greater, with 300–500 and 3000–4000 capillaries mm^{-2} respectively. Most coronary venous drainage (95%) is into the right atrium via the coronary sinus. The rest drains directly into the heart chambers via the thebsian veins.

In the normal heart there is little collateral flow in the coronary circulation and occlusion of a branch will lead to an area of myocardium becoming ischaemic. The coronary arteries thus function as organ end arteries. As the myocardium contracts during systole the transmural pressure on the coronary arterioles rises to systolic pressures. Flow is therefore inhibited during systole and most coronary flow occurs during ventricular diastole, so the coronary flow wave is in antiphase to that of the rest of the circulation. This is particularly the case in the left coronary artery (Figure 5.25). The reduction in flow during systole is exacerbated by low pressure in the sinuses of Valsalva behind the open valve leaflets. The greatest myocardial pressure occurs in the subendocardial or internal layers, making this region the most vulnerable to ischaemia.

Coronary blood flow depends on the A-V pressure difference, the length of diastole, the rate of pressure decay during diastole and the resistance of the myocardial vascular bed. More than any other vascular bed in the body, coronary blood flow depends directly on the O_2 demand of its end organ – the heart. This is because with the very high capillary density, O_2 extraction is nearly maximal even at basal resting flows (Table 5.5).

Therefore the only way the heart can increase its workload is to increase its O_2 supply by increasing coronary flow, and there is an almost linear relationship between increasing O_2 usage and coronary blood flow. As the systemic demand for cardiac output increases, e.g. during exercise, heart rate increases with increased stroke volume and the diastolic interval decreases. Metabolic needs of the work in systole must therefore be largely met by the coronary blood flow in the ever-shortening diastole.

Coronary reserve

During basal flow at rest, coronary blood flow is autoregulated (see Chapter 6) over the normal range of

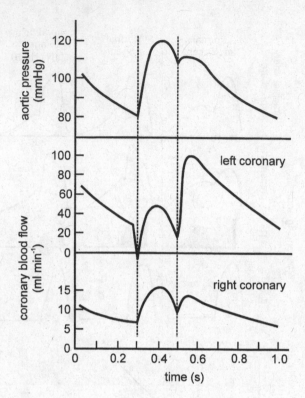

Figure 5.25 – Flow in the coronary arteries compared with changes in aortic pressure over the cardiac cycle.[9]

perfusion pressure, so long as perfusion pressure is more than ~60 mmHg. The difference in flow between basal flow and flow at maximum dilatation for a given perfusion pressure is known as the **coronary blood flow reserve**. It is normally five times the basal flow i.e. 70 rising to 350 ml min^{-1}.

Figure 5.26 shows these features and also the loss in coronary blood flow reserve seen in a hypertrophied heart. This has a larger myocardium which supplies and operates at a higher end-diastolic pressure requiring a greater isovolumic pressure rise. The density of capillaries in the hypertrophied myocardium may also be reduced. Coronary flow reserve may also be reduced by

Table 5.5 – Oxygen budget of the heart

The myocardium extracts 13 ml 100 ml^{-1} blood, i.e. OER = 65%:
- 20% maintains basal metabolic needs of the heart itself
- 0.4% is utilised in cardiac electrical activity
- 80% provides the energy used in pumping blood through the circulation

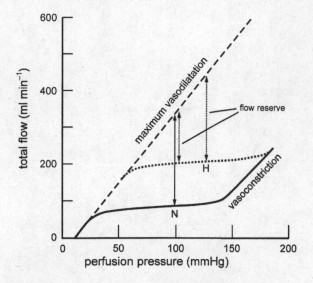

Figure 5.26 – Autoregulation of coronary flow and coronary flow reserve. At basal metabolic rate the normal working point of the heart is shown by 'N' giving a fivefold flow reserve. In a hypertrophied heart (broken line) the basal flow is greater and flow reserve is reduced at normal perfusion pressure. At elevated perfusion pressure it improves (H). Flow appears to fall to zero at 20–40 mmHg due to viscous effects in the microcirculation (adapted from Hoffman 1987).[10]

raised right atrial pressure or reduced aortic diastolic pressure, e.g. through aortic valve regurgitation or aortic stiffening with age, both of which reduce A-V pressure difference, or by reduced O_2 capacity of blood, e.g. anaemia.

Coronary artery stenosis

The most significant impairment to coronary flow is stenotic disease of the coronary arteries. A > 60% diameter stenosis will reduce the basal flow, and as little as 30% stenosis will reduce the flow at maximum dilatation. Flow to the subendocardium is affected the most as extramural pressure restricting the flow is higher towards the inner wall of the left ventricle. A reduction in flow during exercise leads to temporary ischaemia and the patient experiencing the pain of **angina pectoris**. Ischaemia produces a delayed relaxation in cells, so

contraction is impaired. If sufficiently extensive, ventricular performance is then decreased, which will exacerbate the deficit in O_2 supply via the coronary arteries. Severe and prolonged ischaemia leads to infarcts and the patient experiences a heart attack. If a stenosis develops slowly enough, collateral channels may develop to delay the onset of ischaemia.

References

1. Strackee J, Westerhof N. *The Physics of Heart and Circulation*. Bristol: Institute of Physics, 1993.

2. Rowell LB. *Human Cardiovascular Control*. Oxford: Oxford University Press, 1993.

3. Warner HR, Cox A. A mathematical model of heart rate control by sympathetic and vagus efferent information. *Journal of Applied Physiology* 1962; **17**: 349–355.

4. *The New Medicine*, vol. 3: *Cardiology*. Ed. Hamish Watson, MTP Press Ltd: Lancaster 1983.

5. O'Rourke MF. Pressure and flow waves in systemic arteries and the anatomical design of the arterial system. *Journal of Applied Physiology* 1967; **23**: 139–149.

6. Lilly LS (ed.). *Pathophysiology of Heart Disease*. Baltimore: Williams & Wilkins, 1998.

7. Little RC, Little WC. *Physiology of the Heart and Circulation*, 4th edn. Chicago: Year Book, 1989.

8. Nichols WW, O'Rourke MF. *Mcdonald's Blood Flow in Arteries*, 4th edn. London: Arnold, 1998.

9. Berne RM, Levy MN. *Cardiovascular Physiology*, 3rd edn. St Louis: CV Mosby, 1977.

10. Hoffman BB. A critical review of coronary reserve. *Circulation* 1987; **75 (suppl. 1)**: I6–16.

Further reading

Levick JR. *An Introduction to Cardiovascular Physiology*. Oxford: Butterworth-Heinemann, 1995.

Matthews LR. *Cardiopulmonary Anatomy and Physiology*. Philadelphia: Lippincott, 1996.

Walsh C, Wilde P. *Practical Echocardiography*. London: Greenwich Medical Media, 1999.

6

THE CARDIOVASCULAR SYSTEM – THE CIRCULATION

THE CARDIOVASCULAR SYSTEM – THE CIRCULATION

Outline

The chapter describes the structure of the blood vessels. It then shows how control of flow in the circulation is achieved through control of blood pressure, peripheral vascular resistance, the venous reservoir, total vascular volume, and the calf muscle and respiratory pumps. Changes in blood flow on standing and during exercise are examined. The effects of ageing, hypertension and diabetes on the circulation are described, and cerebral and pulmonary and hepatosplanchnic circulations are discussed.

Properties of the circulation

The mean rate of flow and mean pressure drop at various points in the circulation depend upon the vascular resistance of the blood vessels as given by Poiseuille's equation. Figure 6.1 shows the values for a number of parameters around the circulation.

Notes:

- The number of vessels at each level increases towards the periphery.

- The cross-sectional area (hence surface area) is largest at capillary level but the volume of blood in capillaries is just 5% of the total. The vast increase in surface area at the capillary level enables each red blood cell (RBC) to come into contact with the vessel wall where it can exchange oxygen for carbon dioxide with the adjacent tissue.

- Of total blood volume, 67% is in the veins. Because the veins are at low pressure and have very distensible walls, they act as a reservoir and play an important role in regulating cardiac output.

- The vessel diameter decreases significantly at the level of the arterioles. This produces a large pressure drop at arteriolar level where vascular resistance, related to the number of vessels and their diameter, is greatest. This is the r^4 factor in Poiseuille's equation. Arteriole diameter can be varied by autonomic control and it is changes in resistance at this

level that determines regional blood flow to different organs and tissues.

- In stable conditions the volume flow leaving the heart equals the volume flow returning. Therefore at each level of the whole vascular system the volume flow must be constant, although the flow to

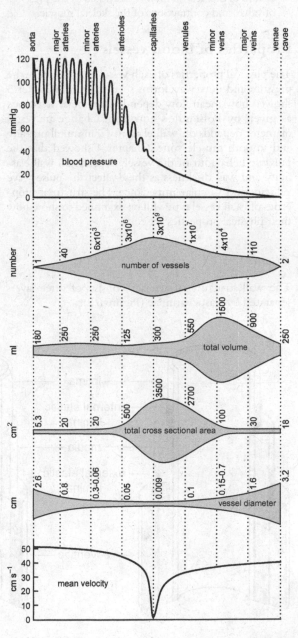

Figure 6.1 – Variation of a number of vessel parameters around the systemic circulation.

individual vascular beds can vary considerably. The blood moving at a lower velocity balances the increase in cross-sectional area in the arterioles, capillaries and venules.

- On the venous side, flow occurs along a relatively modest drop in pressure to the vena cava and right atrium of the heart. This flow is assisted by the presence of valves and contractions of the skeletal muscle.

Properties of blood vessels

The physical properties of each vessel type influence the pressure and flow waveforms seen in them. Chapter 3 showed how mean flow depends on vascular resistance as given by Poiseuille's equation. Change in vessel diameter depends on wall elasticity, transmural pressure and smooth muscle tone. Chapter 4 showed that the pulsatile behaviour of the vessels depends on wall elasticity and wall thickness as these affect the pulse wave velocity and vascular impedance. The structural properties of each vessel type will be examined to show how their physical properties arise.

Arteries

The wall structure of arteries consists of three layers separated by elastic laminae (Figure 6.2).

- **Intima** – innermost layer consisting of **vascular endothelium**. This is a single layer of cells in contact with the blood, backed by a thin layer of elastin and collagen fibres that anchor it to the media. The endothelium responds to many chemical agonists and to shear stress produced by blood flow adjacent to it, to produce **nitric oxide** (endothelium-derived relaxing factor, EDRF). This diffuses into the underlying smooth muscle leading to its relaxation and vasodilatation.

- **Media** – middle layer that makes up the bulk of the vessel wall. This layer is the principal determinant of the vessel's mechanical properties. It is separated from the intima and adventitia by the internal and external elastic laminae respectively. In between these layers are organised layers of a fibrous structure composed of elastin and collagen with layers of smooth muscle fibres running in between. The fibres of the elastin–collagen matrix run circularly round the artery or in a tight helix along the artery. The smooth muscle fibres mostly run parallel to the elastin fibres although some run longitudinally along the vessel. In smaller arteries (< 10 mm diameter) the media is less elastic and contains a higher proportion of muscle cells.

- **Adventitia** – outer-most layer is a strong thick collagen layer with some elastin that merges with

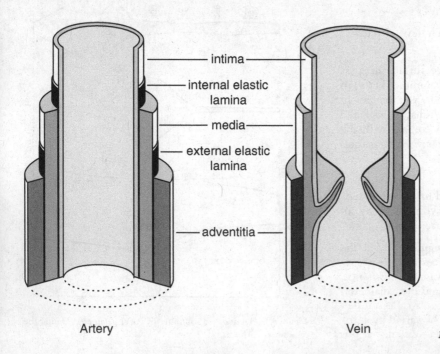

Artery   Vein

Figure 6.2 – Structure of vessel walls.

the surrounding connective tissue thus tethering the artery whilst still allowing considerable movement.

Elastin – as its name suggests elastin is elastic and stretchable. **Collagen** is much stiffer and gives the vessel rigidity under high-pressure loads. In a given vessel, the ratio of elastin to collagen fibres determines how the vessel wall responds to changes in blood pressure over the cardiac cycle. The elastin content allows the vessel wall to stretch when blood pressure increases. The collagen content limits the stretching thereby maintaining the integrity of the vessel wall. This limiting function is seen in the strong collagen layer of the adventitia. Figure 3.47 shows the role of elastin and collagen in the change in aortic diameter as blood pressure increases.

The ratio of elastin to collagen varies significantly between the central and peripheral arteries. In the proximal aorta it is the dominant component with a ratio of 60:40 to collagen. Further down in the abdominal aorta the proportion of elastin decreases and collagen increases and the ratio changes to 30:70. In the peripheral arteries collagen is the dominant component, so vessels get stiffer towards the periphery (Figure 6.3). The role of smooth muscle in the arterial wall is to actively control the diameter of the vessel. Smooth muscle exerts a large effect in smaller arteries and arterioles, but its effect is also present in large arteries.

Atherosclerosis is a disease of muscular arteries in which the intima becomes thickened by fatty deposits

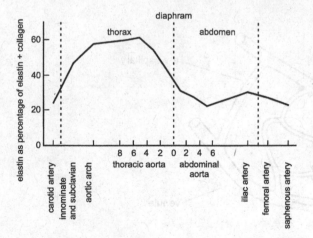

Figure 6.3 – Variation of elastin content in arteries in a dog model (adapted from Harkness *et al.* 1957).[1]

and fibrous tissue to form a plaque. These plaques can have important haemodynamic consequences. Many of the pathological manifestations of this disease result from altered haemodynamics, e.g. stroke, angina and claudication.

The atherosclerotic lesion arises from within the intimal layer of the artery. It starts as fatty streaks, which are typically 1–2 mm wide and up to 10 mm long, formed of foam cells filled with intracellular lipid. These are found in the aorta and coronary arteries in most individuals by 20 years of age. They do not cause symptoms and do not protrude into the arterial lumen.

The next stage in the disease process is the formation of fibrous plaques that appear to develop from fatty streaks. These form an elevated lesion that may protrude into the arterial lumen restricting blood flow to the distal vascular bed. They often contain a necrotic core of cell debris, degenerated foam cells and cholesterol crystals separated from the lumen by a fibrous cap of connective tissue with embedded smooth muscle cells (Figure 6.4). Haemodynamic changes and clinically significant events result from changes in the fibrous plaque as indicated in Table 6.1.

Arterioles

These are small vessels of submillimetre diameter. Their walls are mainly made of smooth muscle and the activity of these muscular walls controls flow to the distal capillary bed. It is at the arteriolar level that the Wormersley parameter α falls to < 1 and flow becomes quasi-steady. These vessels therefore form the terminating resistance at the end of the arterial tree, a resistance that can be varied under autonomic control.

Capillaries

There are two types of capillaries, arteriovenous (A-V) and true capillaries (Figure 6.5).

A-V capillaries – have some muscular coat proximally and can shunt blood to the venules so that it bypasses the tissue bed. They remain open whilst the tissue is at rest.

True capillaries – 0.5–1 mm long and run off the A-V capillaries. Structurally their wall consists of a single layer of endothelial cells 0.5 μm thick. Flow through them is controlled by a sphincter muscle at their origin

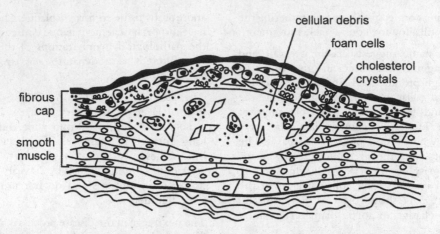

Figure 6.4 – Fibrous plaque in an arterial wall. A necrotic core of cell debris, foam cells and cholesterol crystals is present under a fibrous cap of connective tissue and smooth muscle cells within the intima.[2]

Table 6.1 – Changes occurring in a complicated atherosclerotic lesion

Calcification	leading to vessel rigidity, increasing its fragility and increasing the pulse wave velocity
Haemorrhage into fibrous plaque	resulting in haematoma that further narrows the vessel and may rupture the plaque
Rupture and ulceration	exposing thrombogenic material to the circulating blood
Embolisation	releasing fragments of disrupted atheroma to distal sites
Weakened vessel wall	leading to atrophy and loss of elastic tissue producing vessel dilatation, tortuosity and aneurysm

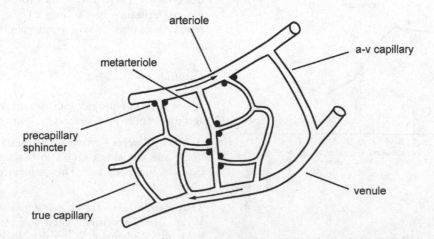

Figure 6.5 – Capillary circulation.

on the A-V capillaries. They anastomose profusely to give the surrounding tissue its blood supply.

The diameter of capillaries (4–7 μm) is smaller than a RBC (8 μm). This means that the RBC has to distort to pass along the capillary. The ratio of surface area to blood volume in capillaries is 6000 cm² for every millilitre of blood filling them. RBC velocity in capillaries is 0.5–1 mm s⁻¹ giving a transit time of 1–2 s. This is more than sufficient to allow the exchange of oxygen and CO_2 with surrounding tissue.

The cellular wall of the capillaries forms a semipermeable membrane with pores through which water, small molecules and ions can freely pass. There is a large exchange of water and low weight molecules diffusing across the capillary wall, but net movement of fluid between blood in the capillaries and extra cellular fluid in surrounding tissue is driven by two forces which together are known as **Starling forces** illustrated in Figure 6.6. The first is the **hydrostatic pressure difference** p, which will tend to drive water out of the capillary and into the tissue. The second force results from the difference in concentration of plasma proteins and sodium ions between the two fluid compartments producing **osmotic pressures** of 17 mmHg and 8 mmHg respectively. These combined

pressures (25 mmHg) form what is known as the **oncotic pressure π**, which tends to drive water into the capillary where concentration is higher.

At the arterial end of the capillary bed, the hydrostatic pressure exceeds the oncotic pressure and there is a net loss of fluid from the capillary into the surrounding tissue space. Due to fluid resistance in the capillary bed there is a drop in hydrostatic pressure, so that at the venous end the oncotic pressure exceeds the hydrostatic pressure. There is then a net flow of fluid from the tissue space back into the capillary. The bulk movement of fluid across the capillary endothelium is 20 lday⁻¹ out of capillaries with 16-18 lday⁻¹ being returned to the blood. The amount of water diffusing between the compartments carrying nutrients, O_2 and CO_2 has been estimated to be 80,000 l/day. Since plasma volume is only 3l, it follows that plasma water is completely exchanged with the interstitial fluid every 3.3 seconds. The interstitial fluid volume is ~ 12 litres.

Lymphatic system

Some plasma proteins do leak into the tissue fluid space and these together with excess fluid are

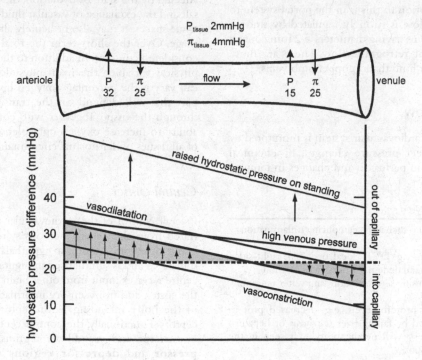

Figure 6.6 – Exchange of fluid across a capillary wall. Transfer into extracellular fluid is given by hydrostatic pressure *p* and transfer into the capillary plasma is driven by oncotic pressure π. The graph shows normal flow (shaded area) out of the capillary at the arteriole end, and back into the capillary at the venule end. The other lines indicate changes under various conditions.

drained from the tissue space by the lymphatic system. The fluid, called **lymph**, moves along the lymphatic vessels towards the thorax where it is returned to the cardiovascular system via the subclavian veins. These travel along the same route as the veins and flow is aided by muscle contractions. The total fluid volume transported in this way amounts to 2–4 litres day^{-1}. A failure in the collection and drainage of lymph leads to a build up of plasma proteins in the tissue fluid space. This reduces the oncotic pressure seen by the capillaries so less fluid returns to the capillaries and the surrounding tissue becomes oedematous (Table 6.2). The rate of fluid transfer into extracellular fluid will also change with hydrostatic pressure in the capillaries (Figure 6.6).

Veins

As with the arteries, three layers may be recognised in the walls of veins, although the media and adventitia are less well defined as separate layers (Figure 6.2). The walls of veins are thin and elastic and are capable of great dilatation. In most vein walls muscle fibres are sparse. One exception to this is in the portal system to the liver where flow is strongly regulated by smooth muscle control. Veins having diameters > 2 mm contain **valves** to prevent retrograde flow. These are more prevalent in lower limb than in upper limb veins.

Control of flow

The state of the cardiovascular system is monitored by sensors that detect pressure changes, biochemical changes, changes in perfusion and changes in temper-

Table 6.2 – Causes of oedema

Arteriolar dilatation – such as is seen during inflammation

Venous obstruction, e.g. DVT (local oedema), right-sided heart failure (general oedema), portal hypertension
Kidney disease – causing severe sodium and water retention

Decreased plasma protein levels, e.g. decreased protein production caused by failing liver (cirrhosis or hepatitis) Increased capillary wall permeability – as seen in the inflammatory response

Blocked lymphatic drainage – increasing protein levels in extravascular tissue space

ature. These feed back to control mechanisms that operate to maintain adequate blood flow to all parts of the body. This forms a complex integrated system that has a considerable degree of redundancy so that if one mechanism of control fails other mechanisms can compensate. Response times vary from seconds for autonomic neural activity, minutes to hours for hormonal activity, to months for responses to chronic changes. Flow to vital organs is maintained by autoregulation mechanisms that effectively prioritise flow to these regions. As conditions change the cardiovascular system responds to maintain its integrity.

The physical variables affecting blood flow that can be controlled are cardiac output, vascular resistance and total blood volume. Cardiac output may be varied to match demand within the constraints already discussed. Change in vascular resistance is produced by changes in smooth muscle tone in all vessels, but in the arterioles in particular. Variable resistance enables flow to be redirected from one part of the system to another and blood pressure and tissue perfusion to be controlled. Constriction on the arterial side is known as **vasoconstriction**, that on the venous side as **venoconstriction**. The total volume of the system is affected by the state of hydration, the concentration of salt and the exchange of vascular fluid with fluid in the tissue spaces. It may also be acutely altered by haemorrhage. Over the short-term the total volume may be considered constant. In addition to the control of these physical variables, the main physiological factor that can vary is the percentage oxygen uptake by tissue. In part this will depend on the transit time of blood through the tissue. Together with control of flow, the ability to increase oxygen uptake ensures the viability of all tissues under normal circumstances.

Central control

Overall control of the cardiovascular system is orchestrated from the central nervous system with control being distributed along a hypothalamic–medullary–spinal axis and is summarised in Figure 6.7. This control centre receives input from other brain centres including the cortex and from sensory information from all parts of the body including baroreceptors and chemoreceptors. Functionally, the control centre includes vasoconstrictor and vasodilator regions, also known as **pressor** and **depressor regions** respectively, and cardio-excitatory and -inhibitory regions. It includes sensors for blood acidity (pH), PO_2 and PCO_2, affecting respiratory as well as cardiovascular control. Total fluid

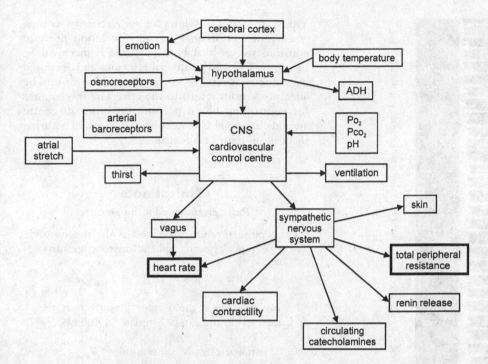

Figure 6.7 – Central control pathways involved in regulating the cardiovascular system. ADH, antidiuretic hormone.

volume is also regulated from the control centre of the brain through the detection of plasma osmolarity and the release of antidiuretic hormone (ADH) and sympathetic outflow to the kidneys. Core temperature is sensed in the hypothalamus and flow to the skin controlled to maintain normal temperature.

Neural control of the peripheral circulation is mainly via the sympathetic nervous system. There is normally a continual outflow of sympathetic impulses to systemic arterioles causing vasoconstriction. Vasodilatation via the parasympathetic nervous system is effected by inhibitory impulses to preganglionic sympathetic neurons in the spinal cord. They therefore cause vasodilatation by modifying the sympathetic outflow rather than by acting directly on the arterioles themselves. Vasodilatation then occurs passively as sympathetic tone is withdrawn. Figure 6.8 shows the effect of changes in sympathetic tone on peripheral arterioles in the foot of a subject in a warm room. The waveforms, taken from the posterior tibial artery, show a characteristic cycling in diastolic flow over 50–60 s as peripheral resistance varies.

Some vasodilatory fibres do travel via the parasympathetic nervous system to act directly on blood vessels. These include the salivary glands and gastric mucosa active in digestion, the skin of the face and neck to cause blushing, and the external genitalia. They work by inhibiting active smooth muscle tone at the end organ site, releasing vasodilatory substances to increase local blood flow. Outflow to the heart consists of sympathetic excitatory fibres and vagal inhibitory fibres.

Input from interacting higher brain centres includes emotions such as fear and anger, stimulating thoughts, thirst, food intake and sexual arousal. Other external inputs that affect the cardiovascular system include pain and ambient temperature. Somatic pain causes tachycardia and hypertension while severe visceral pain causes bradycardia, hypotension and even fainting. Ambient cold causes a rise in blood pressure that increases left ventricular workload and may trigger angina in susceptible patients.

Control of blood pressure and perfusion

Tissue perfusion depends on the A-V pressure difference. The need to maintain adequate perfusion means that arterial blood pressure must be controlled over the physiologic range of conditions.

Mean aortic blood pressure (BP) depends on cardiac output (CO) and total systemic vascular resistance (TVR) as shown in the blood pressure equation:

$$BP = CO \times TVR$$

Blood Pressure Equation

This is analogous to Ohm's law for electricity (voltage = current × resistance). From the blood pressure equation we see that blood pressure is increased by increasing CO and peripheral resistance and decreased by reducing these. To increase CO there must be adequate venous return to the atria. The mechanisms for controlling blood pressure therefore all centre around changes in CO, vascular resistance and ensuring that venous return is adequate.

Clinical note
Pulse pressure and mean pressure

The pulse pressure is defined as the difference between peak systolic and end-diastolic pressures:

$$\text{Pulse pressure} = (P_{\text{systolic}} - P_{\text{diastolic}}).$$

Mean pressure is the average pressure over the cardiac cycle and can be estimated as follows:

$$\text{Central arteries: Mean pressure} \approx P_{\text{diastolic}} + \tfrac{1}{2}\text{ pulse pressure} = \tfrac{1}{2}\,(P_{\text{systolic}} + P_{\text{diastolic}}).$$

$$\text{Peripheral arteries: Mean pressure} \approx P_{\text{diastolic}} + \tfrac{1}{3}\text{ pulse pressure} = \tfrac{1}{3}\,(P_{\text{systolic}} + 2P_{\text{diastolic}}).$$

This takes account of the fact that towards the periphery the pressure wave becomes more pulsatile.

Venous reservoir

The venous system performs an important role in the distribution of flow acting as a reservoir, in what is a closed circuit system with a fixed volume of blood. Table 6.3 shows the distribution of blood in the body at rest. The veins contain 75% of total blood volume with up to one-third of that in the small veins and venules. As discussed in Chapter 3, the transmural pressure over which veins collapse is in the middle of the physiologic range. In addition, the vein wall is more compliant than the arterial wall, the venules being the most compliant part. This means that the volume of the venous space can vary by a large amount with only a small change in fluid pressure (Figure 6.9). Figure 6.10 shows that the venules will experience a larger pressure when the arterioles supplying them are vasodilated and flow is at its greatest.

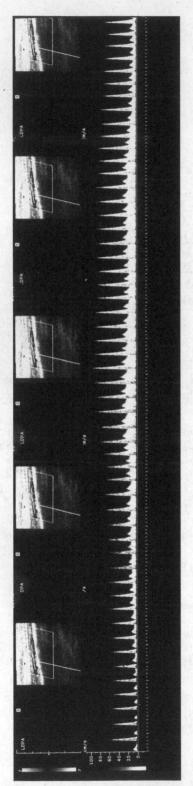

Figure 6.8 – Doppler waveform from the posterior tibial artery of a normal subject in a warm room. It shows a characteristic cycling of the diastolic flow due to sympathetic activity in the peripheral vessels.

Table 6.3 – Typical distribution of blood volume in a 75-kg man at rest[3]

	(ml)		(%)	
Systemic vessels				
Arteries	640	⎫	11.4	⎫
Capillaries	300	⎬ 4860	5.4	⎬ 86.8
Veins	3920	⎭	70.0	⎭
Pulmonary vessels				
Arteries	119	⎫	2.1	⎫
Capillaries	142	⎬ 458	2.5	⎬ 8.2
Veins	197	⎭	3.5	⎭
Heart	282		5.0	
Total	5600		100	

Within the body, the two most compliant regions are the **hepatic–splanchnic circulation**, which includes the liver, gastrointestinal tract, pancreas and spleen, and the **skin circulation**. Both regions are richly innervated so both vaso- and venoconstriction can occur. Consider the case of generalised vasoconstriction of these compliant regions (Figure 6.10a). There is a larger pressure drop across the narrow constricted arterioles so pressure in the post-capillary venules is reduced. This is the r^4 effect of Poiseuille's equation. As the venule pressure drops, the venules collapse and the volume of blood they contained moves into the central veins. In

other words, with vasoconstriction there is a shift in blood volume from the venules and small veins into the central conduit veins. This increases the filling pressure of the right atrium, which in turn results in increased CO, as discussed previously.

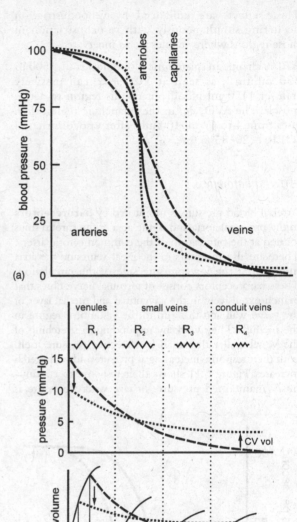

Figure 6.10 – Operation of the venous reservoir: (a) Change in pressure across a capillary bed at rest (solid line), with vasoconstriction (dotted line) and vasodilatation (dashed line). Note that most of the pressure drop occurs at the arteriolar level; (b) the top part shows the changes on the venous side in more detail with the volume–pressure curves at each level shown below. Following vasoconstriction, pressure in the venules drops, the venules collapse and the volume of blood within them moves into the larger conduit veins (CV) returning blood to the heart ((b) from Rowell 1993).[4]

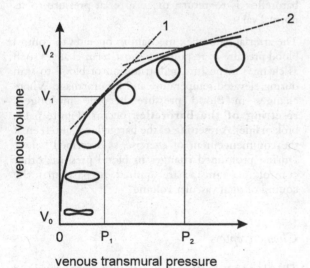

Figure 6.9 – Typical volume–pressure curve of an isolated vein. The broken lines 1 and 2 show the compliance ($\Delta V/\Delta P$) at two transmural pressures, P_1 and P_2. Note that compliance is greater at lower pressures. V_0 is the unstressed volume, which is the volume at zero transmural pressure. The change in volume from V_1 to V_2 is the passive effect of increasing the pressure. Such a pressure increase will occur when there is arteriole dilatation increasing flow into the venules.[4]

The opposite effect occurs when there is generalised vasodilatation. Pressure in the post-capillary veins increases and so they distend, increasing their volume thereby reducing central venous volume, right atrial filling pressure and CO.

These effects are enhanced by venoconstriction occurring simultaneously with vasoconstriction in those regions where venules are so innervated.

A 70% change in splanchnic blood flow from 1500 to 350 mlmin^{-1}, as seen at $\dot{V}O_2$ *max*, can passively transfer 1150 ml blood out of this region to active muscle. The AVO$_2$ *diff* in the splanchnic region then rises from 4 to 17 ml 100 ml^{-1} after vasoconstriction (OER = 20–85%).

Arterial baroreflex

Arterial blood pressure is monitored by **baroreceptors** in the proximal aorta and in the area of the carotid sinus located at the bifurcation of the common carotid artery. There are also receptors in the great veins and the atria monitoring the low-pressure side of the circulation. These baroreceptors consist of terminal nerve fibres that branch extensively in the adventitial and medial layer of the vessel wall and that run to the vasomotor region in the medulla. They work by responding to stretching of the vessel wall rather than by detecting pressure itself, with their response increasing as pressure and wall stretch increases. Figure 6.11 shows their response to continuously maintained pressure. *In vivo* where pressure is

pulsatile, their firing rate is also increased by the rate of increasing change in pressure as well as by the mean pressure. Thus their firing rate increases during the systolic rise in pressure and falls in the falling post-systolic phase. It acts as a proportional–differential sensor. Baroreceptor output therefore conveys information about mean arterial pressure, the amplitude of pulse pressure and the steepness of the pressure rise, and hence includes information about heart rate and contratility.

The baroreflex forms a negative feedback loop in which increased neural activity from the baroreceptor due to raised pressure leads to a lowering of heart rate and myocardial contractility, thereby reducing cardiac output. Vasoconstrictor tone in the periphery is also reduced to decrease arterial pressure. The opposite occurs when arterial pressure drops and baroreceptor activity decreases. Peripheral arterioles are vasoconstricted. Pressure in the venous reservoir drops and blood moves into the great veins where increased heart rate and cardiac contractility move blood toward the arterial side, so raising arterial pressure. The main baroreceptors controlling arterial pressure are those in the carotid sinus, and for this reason these responses are known as the **carotid sinus reflex**. Low pressure at the carotid sinus also stimulates the release of renin, as described below. The overall effect of the carotid sinus baroreflex is to return mean arterial pressure to its normal value.

The arterial baroreflex mechanism operates to control blood pressure in response to short-term changes such as changes in posture, redistribution of blood to skin during elevated temperature and haemorrhage. Where changes in blood pressure become prolonged, **resetting of the baroreflex** occurs (Figure 6.11, broken line). A resetting of the baroreflex is also seen at the commencement of exercise, as described below. During prolonged changes in blood pressure, other control mechanisms are applied, in particular the control of total vascular volume.

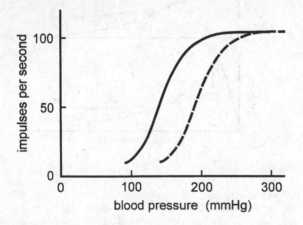

Figure 6.11 – Nervous output of the carotid sinus baroreceptors as a function of sinus blood pressure (solid line). The broken line shows the effect of resetting the baroreceptor reflex response (adapted from Landgren 1952).[5]

Chemoreceptors

The blood levels of oxygen, carbon dioxide and blood pH are sensed at several places in the circulation. Within the capillary bed of end organ tissues they provide a stimulus for local control of blood flow ensuring that adequate perfusion and clearance of metabolites is maintained. Within the brain there is very strong control of systemic and cerebral blood flow in response to changes in blood gases and pH.

In addition the partial pressure of oxygen PO_2 and blood pH are sensed in the **carotid and aortic bodies**. These are adjacent to the carotid bifurcation and on the aortic arch respectively. They are very small vascular organs with a large blood flow and high metabolic rate. Sensory nerve fibres from these bodies run to the cardiovascular and respiratory centres in the brain. In normal subjects they play little or no role in the control of ventilation. They only become significant when a reduction in $PO_2 < 50–60$ mmHg (normally 100 mmHg) leads to an increase in pulmonary ventilation and sympathetic outflow.

CATECHOLAMINES

Adrenaline (epinephrine) and **noradrenaline** (norepinephrine) are two hormones that have an important influence on the cardiovascular system. Together they are known as **catecholamines**. They are released into the bloodstream from the adrenal medulla, situated adjacent to the upper pole of the kidney, by sympathetic stimulation. There they are produced in the ratio of 80% adrenaline to 20% noradrenaline. Noradrenaline is also the neurotransmitter produced by the sympathetic nerve synapses controlling vascular tone. At these synapses the concentration of noradrenaline is very much higher than in the general circulation. Where sympathetic nerves are very active there can be spillover from the synapses into the bloodstream, otherwise noradrenaline is removed or reabsorbed at the synapses fairly quickly. The actions of these hormones depend on the type of receptors present in each part of the circulation. Their action is further modified by locally produced substances such as metabolites that amplify or diminish their effect.

There are two kinds of receptors, α and β, together known as **adrenergic receptors** since they respond to adrenaline and noradrenaline. As the sympathetic nerves release noradrenaline, the nerve fibres are called **adrenergic nerves**. Adrenaline and noradrenaline both bind to **α-receptors** to produce an increase in heart rate and cardiac contractility, and vasoconstriction in the peripheral arterioles and the splanchnic and cutaneous veins. This produces an increase in total peripheral resistance and a rise in mean blood pressure. The rise in blood pressure is sensed by the baroreceptors and reflex vagal bradycardia is produced, so overall cardiac output is slightly reduced.

Adrenaline also binds to **β-receptors** whereas noradrenaline has very little affinity for them. Stimulation of β-receptors causes an increase in heart rate and cardiac contractility and vasodilatation of the peripheral arterioles in skeletal muscle. So long as venous return is sufficient, this produces an increase in cardiac output and an increase in systolic blood pressure, but a lowering of diastolic pressure as total peripheral resistance is reduced.

At the blood levels normally produced by stimulation of the adrenal medulla, adrenaline has a greater effect on β- than α-receptors, so the normal response to its release is vasodilatation of skeletal muscle. This together with its effects of increased cardiac output, constriction of the splanchnic and cutaneous circulations so moving blood from the venous reservoir, increased rate and depth of breathing, and increased release of metabolic fuels prepares the body to respond to stress such as 'fight or flight'.

Figure 6.12 shows the effect of adrenaline and noradrenaline on peripheral resistance in skeletal muscle. At lower concentrations of adrenaline there is a vasodilator effect as β-receptors are stimulated. However, at higher concentrations the net effect is of a vasoconstrictor as both α- and β-receptors are stimulated. However, the overall resistance is still less than when noradrenaline from the sympathetic nerves stimulates the β-receptors alone.

Drugs that block the α- and β-receptors are used to control the effects of their stimulation when that is deleterious in a patient with heart disease.

Autoregulation

Autoregulation is the ability of an organ to maintain blood flow, for a given metabolic rate, within a narrow range over a wide range of changes in perfusion pressure. Examples of such organs are myocardium, kidney, brain and placenta. This control is independent of the central nervous system and depends on local conditions such as locally produced vasodilator substances and the response to local vessel stretching caused by increases in perfusion pressure. The response time to sudden changes in perfusion pressure is typically 30–60 s. Autoregulation stabilises both tissue perfusion and capillary filtration pressure that affect fluid loss into extravascular tissue. Its effect is shown in Figure 6.13.

Outside the autoregulated range flow follows changes in pressure and in the case of low pressure this may cause ischaemic injury. Local control within a tissue is also affected by chemical changes such as partial oxygen and carbon dioxide pressures (PO_2, PCO_2), blood acidity pH, circulating hormones and metabolic products.

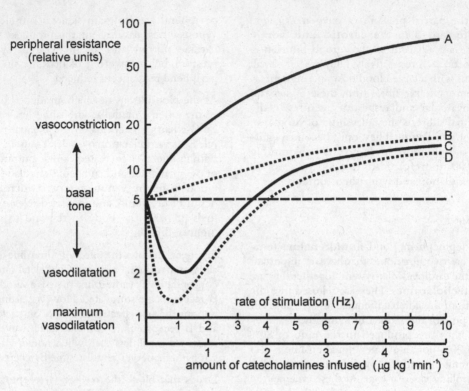

Figure 6.12 – Change in vascular resistance of skeletal muscle with adrenergic stimulation, with stimulation of sympathetic vasoconstrictor fibres (A), noradrenaline infusion (B), stimulation of adrenal medulla (C) and adrenaline infusion (D).[6,7]

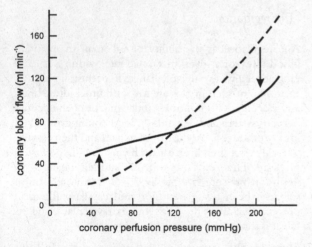

Figure 6.13 – Autoregulation of coronary flow in an animal model. Perfusion pressure was abruptly increased or decreased from a control level at the point where the two lines cross. Immediately after, the intervention flow was that shown by the broken line. As the autoregulation mechanisms took effect flow reached a steady-state on the solid line. This experiment demonstrates autoregulation over 60–180 mmHg.[7,8]

Metabolic hyperaemia

Metabolic hyperaemia is the increase in blood flow seen in exercising skeletal muscle and myocardium. This may be initiated by changes in sympathetic tone and by locally produced vasodilator substances produced in response to increased flow. Greater flow increases endothelial wall shear stress which stimulates the release of nitric oxide (endothelium-derived relaxing factor, EDRF). This diffuses directly into the underlying smooth muscle causing dilatation of the vessels. Such flow-induced vasodilation affects all the proximal arteries including the main supply arteries. For example, hyperaemia in the forearm can increase brachial artery diameter by up to 50%. There is thus a matching of reduced vascular resistance in the supply vessels to the dilated arterioles in the distal vascular bed. This increase in flow required by active muscle resets the working point of autoregulation, as shown for coronary flow in a dog in Figure 6.14.

Notes:

- At any given metabolic rate flow is controlled within a narrow range by autoregulation.

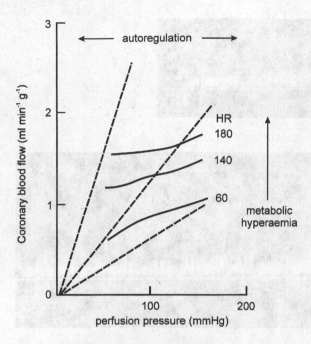

Figure 6.14 – Effect of perfusion pressure and metabolic rate on coronary flow in a dog. Broken lines show the theoretical pressure–flow relationship at constant resistance. The steepest line has lowest resistance. Solid lines show actual variation in flow at three heart rates as autoregulation occurs. The increase in flow with heart rate is metabolic hyperaemia.[9]

- The broken lines indicate the theoretical increase in flow with increasing pressure if flow resistance remained constant. Lowest resistance is the steepest line.

- As metabolic rate increases the autoregulated flow also increases.

Reactive hyperaemia

If blood flow to a region is restricted for a short time, then upon release of the restriction, flow is increased at first and then falls exponentially back to normal levels. This is called reactive hyperaemia and may be seen following occlusion of a limb with an inflated cuff. When the occlusion is > 3 min, vasodilatation of the distal vascular bed will be near maximal and the increased flow restores the oxygen and nutrient deficiency suffered by the tissue as rapidly as possible. Where occlusion has been lengthy (> 1 h) as during some surgical procedures, instead of a hyperaemic reaction blood flow falls to abnormally low levels within minutes

of reperfusion. This is caused by the build up of free radicals during the ischaemic period. The result is that they damage the tissue and capillary walls causing leukocyte adhesion and obstruction. This phenomenon is known as **ischaemia–reperfusion injury**.

Figure 6.15 shows reactive hyperaemia in the hand following release of a clenched fist. During fist clench (a) the peripheral vessels in the hand form a very high-resistance and diastolic flow is abolished. The fingers become blanched as the blood pool is squeezed out and not replaced. Upon fist release, the arterioles in the hand dilate and the skin flushes as the vessels respond to the temporary oxygen deficit. Recovery to normal resting flows occurs over 45 s in this example.

Control of vascular volume

Control of the total volume of the cardiovascular system is closely related to overall control of extracellular fluid. **Extracellular fluid** includes **interstitial fluid** and the **circulating plasma volume**. The mechanisms involved are summarised in Figure 6.16.

Glomerular filtration

Within the kidney fluid and salt levels are regulated by a process of ultrafiltration out of the bloodstream into nephrons, followed by selective reabsorption along the tubule of the nephron (Figure 6.17). There are 1–1.5 million nephrons in each kidney. Renal blood flow is 1.1 l min⁻¹ containing a plasma volume of 600 ml min⁻¹. Filtration occurs in Bowman's capsule where the filtrate is collected from the glomerulus, a knot of capillaries. The process involves Starling forces (Figure 6.6) but blood pressure is maintained at a higher level than in a normal capillary bed (45 and 32 mmHg respectively) by the fact that the arteriole leaving the glomerulus is smaller than that entering. The volume of filtrate amounts to 125 ml min⁻¹ or 180 l day⁻¹ carrying 1100 g sodium chloride and other solutes. Since normal plasma volume is ~3 litres, it is clear that the plasma is filtered and reabsorbed in the tubules many times a day.

Antidiuretic hormone

Extracellular fluid volume is closely controlled to maintain its osmolarity, which mainly depends on sodium concentration (Na⁺). **Osmoreceptors** in the

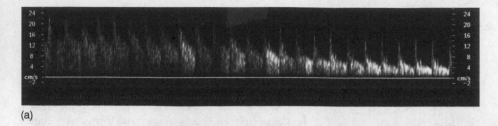

(a)

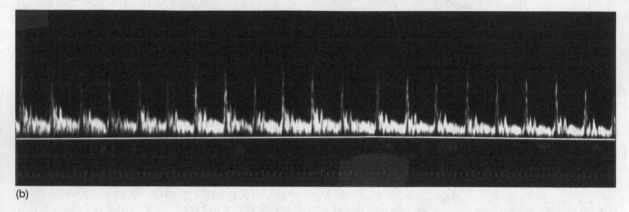

(b)

Figure 6.15 – Doppler waveforms from a radial artery showing reactive hyperaemia in the hand. (a) Flow during the holding of a clenched fist; (b) flow upon fist release showing hyperaemic flow and recovery to the resting flow.

anterior hypothalamus of the brain sense the osmolarity of plasma and alter the level of antidiuretic hormone (ADH) (or vasopressin) released by the pituitary, to maintain the osmolarity of plasma at normal levels. ADH controls the volume of water excreted by the kidneys. For example, ingestion of salt or water deficiency raises plasma osmolarity and increases ADH release, whilst excessive fluid ingestion suppresses ADH

release. This response occurs within minutes of a change in osmolarity being detected. Control of Na^+ levels is effected by angiotensin II and aldosterone, which both increase Na^+ reabsorption by the kidneys. Atrial natriuretic peptide increases Na^+ excretion. These mechanisms are normally adequate to maintain the circulating plasma volume. However, maintenance of circulating volume will take precedence over

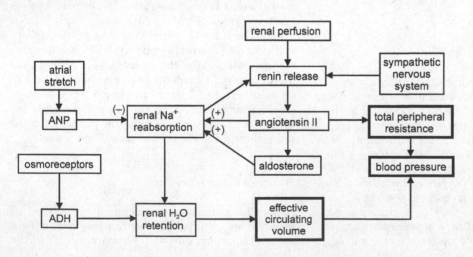

Figure 6.16 – Factors controlling total blood volume. ANP, atrial natriuretic peptide; ADH, antidiuretic hormone.

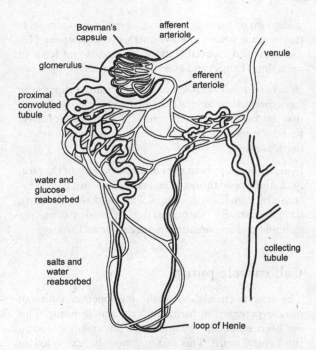

Figure 6.17 – A nephron. Note that the afferent arteriole to the glomerulus is larger than the efferent arteriole so that pressure in the glomerulus is higher than in the distal capillary network. Each kidney contains 1–1.5 million nephrons.

osmotic regulation to ensure survival. For example, ingestion of water together with haemorrhage will lead to a reduction in diuresis to maintain plasma volume even though osmolarity will then be reduced.

Renin–angiotensin–aldosterone system

This is an important mechanism for controlling total blood volume and blood pressure. It also affects fluid transfer between capillaries and extracellular fluid. It is triggered when plasma volume or blood pressure is low and acts to increase them.

The process begins with the release of the enzyme renin from the kidney where it acts on the angiotensin precursor from which the hormone angiotensin II is formed. Renin persists in the blood for ~30 min. The primary controller of renin release in humans is sympathetic activity, arising in response to the arterial baroreceptors, acting on the glomerular arterioles in the kidney. It is also released by a reduction in pressure distending the afferent arterioles in the kidney, such as occurs when there is renal artery stenosis. Reduction in

sodium concentration in the kidney tubule causes renin release as well.

Angiotensin II persists in the blood for ~1 min and has a number of effects. First, it is a powerful vasoconstrictor that acts directly on smooth muscle by reinforcing activity from the sympathetic nervous system. It also acts on the brain to modify the arterial baroreflex control of the heart by inhibiting vagal outflow. Angiotensin II therefore acts to increase blood pressure by enhancing sympathetic vasoconstriction whilst at the same time suppressing reflex vagal bradycardia in the heart. Second, it stimulates the release of the hormone aldosterone from the adrenal cortex. Angiotensin II also affects the central nervous system to provoke water ingestion, increased sodium ingestion and secretion of antidiuretic hormone (ADH).

Aldosterone increases the reabsorption of sodium by the kidney. A higher sodium content in plasma increases plasma volume by causing reabsorption of extravascular fluid into the circulation. The effects of aldosterone are much slower to develop and act much longer than those of angiotensin II. Thus the renin–angiotensin–aldosterone system acts in both short- and long-term control of arterial blood pressure regulation.

Atrial baroreflex

Changes in circulating volume are detected by stretch receptors in the right and left atria. When the atria are stretched by increased venous pressure they release **atrial natriuretic peptide** which acts to increase sodium and water excretion by the kidneys and reduce blood pressure. It does this by reducing renin release, inhibiting aldosterone, reducing peripheral vascular resistance, reducing cardiac output and increasing the transduction of plasma water into the interstitial space. In response to the atrial stretch receptors there is a rapid alteration in urine flow. By these means it reduces blood pressure and circulating volume.

Skin flow and temperature control

The skin circulation has the important function of allowing body temperature to be regulated by moving blood at core temperature to or from the skin surface where heat exchange with the environment can take place. The hypothalamus senses blood temperature and receives information from thermal sensors in the skin. A change in temperature of 0.4°C in the blood bathing the anterior hypothalamus evokes responses to correct it.

The skin is a large organ comprising 39% of normal body mass typical surface area 1.8 m². Using estimated flows, at rest it receives 200–500 ml min⁻¹ blood. When maximally dilated by whole-body heating it may receive as much as 7–8 l min⁻¹. It also acts as a large capacitance that can shift some 1000 ml into or out of circulation.[10]

Skin circulation is of two types. The first is a superficial arteriolar–capillary–venous network that is similar to other peripheral circulations except that it has a prominent collection of subcutaneous venous plexuses. The second type is a series of coiled anastomotic vessels of relatively large diameter with a muscular wall structure in the skin of the fingers, toes, palms of hands and face. These can shunt blood directly from arterioles to venules and act as heat exchangers between warm blood from the core and the cool skin surface. They are under the control of local metabolic factors and the sympathetic nervous system. Normally they have a high level of resting tone and this is withdrawn to open the vessels up. Parasympathetic stimulation of **sweat glands** increases cooling by evaporation at the skin surface and releases a locally acting vasodilator.

Apart from any pigmentation, normal **skin colour** results from the amount and colour of haemoglobin in the cutaneous capillaries. There is usually sufficient oxyhaemoglobin present with its red colour to produce the normal skin colour. If the concentration of reduced haemoglobin is increased to ≥ 5 g 100 ml⁻¹, the skin will turn a blue-purple colour known as **cyanosis**. This may be due, for example, to reduced availability of O_2 or increased O_2 extraction by the tissues. If flow to the skin is so poor that O_2 extraction in the skin capillaries is increased, the skin will turn a pale grey.

Blood vessels in the skin may become overly sensitive to neural vasoconstrictive influences leading to severe vasospasm of the skin vessels at normal room temperatures such as is seen in **Raynaud's phenomenon**. This phenomenon especially affects the hands and leads to pain, skin changes and even tissue necrosis.

Where chronic ischaemia results from sympathetic vasoconstriction at the arteriolar level, the symptoms may be relieved by performing a **sympathectomy**, thereby removing the vasoconstriction due to sympathetic outflow.

Sympathetic supply to the cutaneous vessels of the face, neck and upper thorax is especially sensitive to modulation by higher brain centres. This produces **blushing** or alternatively vasoconstriction and pallor, for example due to embarrassment, or fear and anxiety.

Calf muscle pump

The venous circulation in the leg together with calf muscle contraction form the calf muscle pump. This has been called the 'second heart', returning blood to the central veins. This analogy may be extended in some detail (Table 6.4).

The calf muscle pump function is shown in Figure 6.18. In the normal circulation, venous circulation of the leg is filled via the arteries through the capillary bed. The venous circulation consists of two parts. **The superficial venous system** just below the skin and superficial to the muscle mass includes the long and short saphenous veins. The **deep venous system** lying within the muscle mass includes the tibial and gastrocnemius veins running into the popliteal vein. There are also large valveless venous spaces within the soleal and gastrocnemious muscles called **venous sinuses**. These are 'U'-shaped spaces with both ends emptying towards the heart. The superficial and deep systems are connected by communicating or perforating veins that

Table 6.4 – Comparison of the calf muscle pump and the heart

Calf muscle pump	Heart
Superficial veins supply deep venous space in muscles	Atrium supplies ventricle
Incompetent perforator valves	Incompetent A-V valves
Reflux in LSV and SSV so blood recirculates	A-V shunt via septal defect
Calf DVT reduces muscle venous space	Reduced end-diastolic volume/ventricular filling
Femoral-iliac DVT produces retrograde increase in pressure	Aortic/pulmonary valve stenosis increases ventricular pressure
Muscle weakness	Heart failure

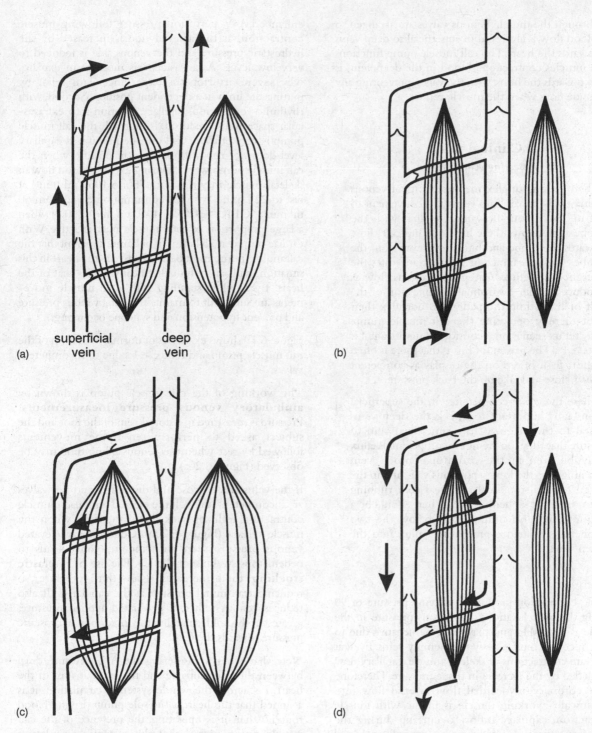

Figure 6.18 – Function of the calf muscle pump in the normal subject. (a) Compression by muscles: blood is propelled centrally with no reflux in the perforators. (b) Relaxation of muscles: valves prevent reflux and veins refill slowly via arterial route. And in a subject with both superficial and deep vein incompetence: (c) incompetent perforators allow blood to leak into the superficial veins during compression. (d) Veins rapidly refill as the same blood refluxes past incompetent valves.

pass through the muscle. Venous valves are arranged so that blood flow is always from superficial to deep veins and towards the heart. The calf muscle pump functions as the muscles contract and blood in the deep veins is driven towards the heart with the valves preventing any retrograde flow when the muscle relaxes.

Clinical note
Assessing venous reflux

When making duplex measurements of venous reflux in the lower limb veins, it is convenient to set up the colour-flow map so that with the probe angled toward the head, red indicates flow towards the probe and blue, flow away from the probe. The appearance of red then indicates the presence of reflux. Antegrade venous flow is produced either by manual compression of the calf or by getting the patient to dorsiflex their foot thereby operating the calf muscle pump. Any reflux seen is only considered significant if it lasts > 1 s. The reason for this is that there is often a short flash of red on the display as competent valves close and take up the back pressure.

Where there is incompetence in the superficial veins it is important to check the deep veins distal to the origin of the superficial vein to ensure that they too are not incompetent. Reflux may be seen in the common femoral vein running into the long saphenous vein, and in the distal femoral-proximal popliteal vein running into the short saphenous vein. There should be a competent valve immediately below the two saphenous junctions preventing reflux into the deep veins.

Muscle contraction produces a driving pressure of 90 mmHg. Upon relaxation, the venous pressure in the muscle is 0 mmHg and may even be negative due to elastic recoil of muscle away from empty veins. Even at moderate contractions of skeletal muscle, capillary flow is impeded by the increase in tissue pressure. Therefore, as for coronary–myocardial flow, arterial flow into rhythmically working muscle is phasic with muscle contraction, capillary inflow occurring during the relaxation phase. In addition to propelling blood towards the heart, calf muscle contractions have two other beneficial effects. The first is enhanced flow into the muscle during exercise. This results from the enhanced A-V perfusion pressure following muscle contraction, as the arterial side is increased by the hydrostatic pressure and the venous side is reduced to very low levels. As an aside, this mechanism explains why severe arteriopaths experience pain relief by putting the limb in a dependent position. Second, with rhythmic contraction, capillary filtration into extravascular space is also reduced. In normals the calf muscle pump is very efficient and oncotic pressure at capillary level does not rise with an upright posture when the calf muscle pump works. During exercise blood flow in skeletal muscle may rise from 750 to 1000 ml min^{-1} at rest to 22 l min^{-1} with O_2 consumption rising from 60 ml min^{-1} (OER = 30%) to 4000 ml min^{-1} (90%) when a large proportion of total muscle bulk is active. With cardiac output at 25 l min^{-1} it becomes apparent that the calf muscle pump must be as effective as the heart in this situation, with an output that nearly equals that of the heart. Even while standing still, small muscle movements are sufficient to maintain central venous pressure and prevent hypotension and syncope occurring.

Figure 6.19 shows examples of normal operation of the calf muscle pump and reflux > 1 s due to incompetent valves.

The working of the calf muscle pump is shown by **ambulatory venous pressure measurements**. Pressure is measured in a dorsal vein of the foot and the subject asked to perform ten tiptoe movements followed by rest when the venous filling time may be observed (Figure 6.20a).

If the veins are varicose and distended, and the valves are incompetent, the volume ejected with each muscle contraction refluxes back down the limb when the muscle relaxes (Figure 6.20b). Continuously elevated venous pressure seen with incompetence leads to oedematous swelling of the leg. The use of an **elastic stocking** then increases tissue fluid pressure, so reducing transmural pressure at the capillaries. It also reduces venous reflux. A graduated applied pressure, greatest at the ankle, matches the increase in hydrostatic pressure towards the feet.

Note that when considering the A-V pressure drop between the left ventricle and the right atrium of the heart, i.e. across the whole systemic circulation, it is assumed that the heart is the sole pump driving blood round. When it is operating, the presence of the calf muscle pump means that the systemic circulation should really be considered as two circuits in series, with the calf muscle pump raising the fluid pressure a second time in its course round the circuit.

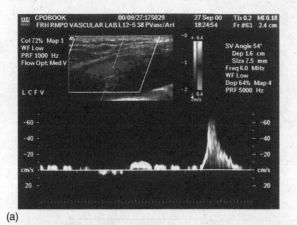

(a)

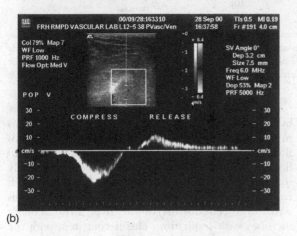

(b)

Figure 6.19 – (a) Doppler waveform of normal phasic flow in the femoral vein followed by a dorsiflexion of the foot showing the operation of the calf muscle pump; (b) Doppler waveform from the popliteal vein showing venous reflux following manual compression of the calf in a patient with deep venous incompetence.

Hepatic–splanchnic circulation

In addition to acting as a functional reservoir for the whole circulation, the hepatic–splanchnic circulation plays an important role in maintenance of cardiac output through the **respiratory pump**. This circulation includes the liver, gastrointestinal tract, pancreas and spleen. The liver receives 25% of its blood flow from the hepatic artery and 75% from the portal vein. The portal vein is supplied from the superior mesenteric artery through the gut, and from the spleen, the pancreas and the gall bladder. The portal vein leads to a capillary bed within the liver, so the blood flowing through this system passes through two capillary networks. There are no valves in the adult portal vein.

Flow in the superior mesenteric artery varies considerably between fasting and following a meal, with volume flow typically increasing from 500 ml min^{-1} during fasting to 1300 ml min^{-1} following a meal. Stenosis of the coeliac trunk and superior mesenteric artery causes mesenteric ischaemia with potentially fatal consequences. In susceptible patients, the increased demand for blood following a meal may produce post-prandial angina.

Both portal vein circulation and hepatic artery circulation drain via the hepatic veins. As a whole, the hepatic–splanchnic circulation contains ~20–25% of total blood volume (1200–1500 ml) and receives ~25% of resting cardiac output (1500 ml min^{-1}). The liver has a very high specific compliance of 25 ml kg^{-1}mmHg^{-1} and effectively acts as a large capacitor adjacent to the right atrium. It typically contains 400 ml blood. In normal liver parenchyma there is no connective tissue scaffolding surrounding the small venules and they easily collapse with an increase in external pressure.

Respiratory pump

Continuity of venous return to the heart is aided by the respiratory pump involving blood flow into the abdominal inferior vena cava (IVC) and venous return from the hepatic–splanchnic circulation. The pump mechanism results from the changes in thoracic and abdominal pressures during the respiratory cycle (Figure 6.21).

During inspiration pressure in the thorax decreases as the rib cage expands and the diaphragm descends into the abdominal cavity. Simultaneously the muscles of the abdominal wall relax. The downward movement of the diaphragm quickly follows this so that there is an overall increase in pressure within the abdominal cavity. This sequence of events produces an increase in pressure gradient along the IVC so that there is an increase in flow from the abdominal IVC towards the heart. The increase in abdominal pressure might also be expected to compress the liver and increase hepatic venous flow. However, the effect of the pressure of the diaphragm on the liver is to collapse the unsupported venules within the liver so preventing hepatic outflow. Flow within the portal vein decreases during this phase but does not actually stop, so hepatic filling continues and the liver increases in volume. When expiration occurs, pressure difference along the IVC is very low so there is almost no flow in the abdominal IVC. As the diaphragm

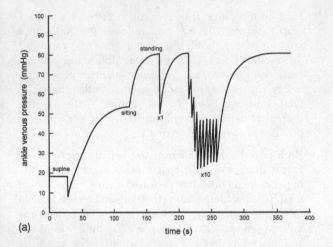

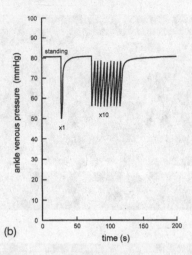

Figure 6.20 – Recorded results of measurements made of ankle venous pressure in (a) a normal subject and (b) a subject with deep venous incompetence. Results for the normal subject show the increase in hydrostatic pressure as the subject sits up and then stands from a supine position. He then performed a single tiptoe dorsiflexion of the foot, operating the calf muscle pump, and then ten consecutive dorsiflexions. Note how the muscle compartment is then fully emptied and refills slowly via the arterial supply. When there is deep vein incompetence (b) the muscle compartment never fully empties and rapidly refills with refluxing blood.

recoils, pressure is relieved on the liver and hepatic outflow recommences providing venous filling to the right atrium. Measurements in dogs have shown that whilst slightly smaller than the IVC flow during inspiration, the increase in liver volume and outflow during expiration closely matches the filling requirement of the thoracic IVC during this phase. Thus there are two phasic flows into the thoracic IVC 180° out of phase with each other. During expiration the abdominal IVC refills with inflow from the lower limbs via the iliac veins, which in turn show a phasicity, with decreased flow during inspiration.

Compression and decompression of the hepatic venules produces a sustained return to the right atrium during expiration. This prevents extreme swings in cardiac output that would occur if the liver and the thoracic IVC both increased their flow during the increase in abdominal pressure during inspiration. In some pathological conditions, for example following trauma, the descent of the diaphragm is impaired. Flow from the liver will then be in phase with the thoracic IVC flow and venous return to the heart will drop significantly during expiration. In patients with cirrhosis of the liver, the liver parenchyma becomes more rigid leading to a reduction in the total hepatic flow from 1300 to 450 ml min^{-1}. Pressure in the portal vein is normally 5–10 mmHg. An increase to > 10 mmHg leads to the development of collaterals from the portal system to the systemic veins that

bypass the liver. Hepatic disease other than cirrhosis may also cause portal hypertension. The reduction of flow through the liver is reflected in reduced forward flow in the portal vein. In some patients it is totally static with only an oscillatory to and fro motion with respiration seen. In the most severe cases of cirrhosis with advanced fibrosis of the liver, flow actually increases with inspiration. This is consistent with the hepatic venules no longer collapsing during inspiration due to the increased rigidity of the organ, resulting in a chronic failure of the respiratory pump. The cardiovascular system responds to the large swings in venous return by expanding total blood volume, reducing peripheral resistance and increasing cardiac output in order to increase IVC pressure and maintain venous return to the heart throughout the respiratory cycle. This **hyperdynamic state** is typical of patients with advanced cirrhosis. High pressure in the gut and portal vein results in the formation of ascites. Examples of portal and hepatic vein flow are shown in Figure 6.22.

There is normally some variation in right and left ventricular output as the pressure in the pulmonary circuit changes with breathing. This is known as **sinus arrhythmia** and is particularly noticeable in children and young adults. It is caused by phasic changes in vagal stimulation producing bradycardia during expiration and tachycardia during inspiration. This is partly a reflex generated by stretch receptors in the

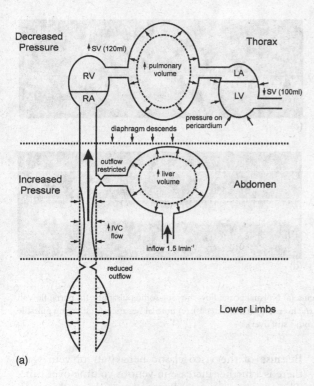

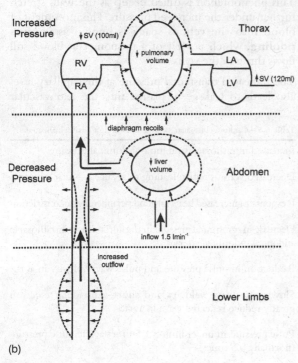

Figure 6.21 – Respiratory pump: (a) during inspiration; (b) during expiration.

lung, but it also arises from control by the brainstem. Tachycardia during inspiration helps to counteract the effect of reduced left ventricular stroke volume due to reduced filling pressure. These effects are seen in Figure 6.23.

Valsalva manoeuvre

The Valsalva manoeuvre is achieved by performing a forced exhalation against a closed glottis. The effects of a Valsalva are shown in Table 6.5. It is sometimes used clinically to induce particular haemodynamic flow conditions to demonstrate or eliminate pathology. The reduction in cardiac output simulates the effects of shock and heart failure. A Valsalva is used in the investigation of the femoral vein flow to halt the normal phasic flow with respiration and to demonstrate the patency of the iliac veins. Figure 6.24a shows how a Valsalva abolishes phasic flow in the common femoral vein leaving just a small cardiac component of flow resulting from the changes in venous pressure as the right atrium relaxes. Figure 6.24b shows how the Valsalva simulates the effects of heart failure on arterial flow with tachycardia and low stroke volume.

Müller manoeuvre

This is the opposite manoeuvre to the Valsalva in which inhalation is performed against a closed glottis. The effects are the opposite to those shown in Table 6.5 with transmural pressure across the aorta being increased. It therefore simulates the effect of arterial stiffening from age or hypertension.

Orthostasis

When we change position from reclining to standing the changes in hydrostatic pressure have significant effects on the circulation. When lying supine, all parts of the body are approximately at the same level as the right atrium and hydrostatic differences are negligible. On standing there is an immediate increase in positive hydrostatic pressure for all points below the heart and negative pressure for points above the heart: in this position 75% of total blood volume lies below the heart. Hydrostatic pressure at the feet is typically 100 mmHg whilst that at the top of the head is −40 mmHg. This negative pressure above the heart is within the

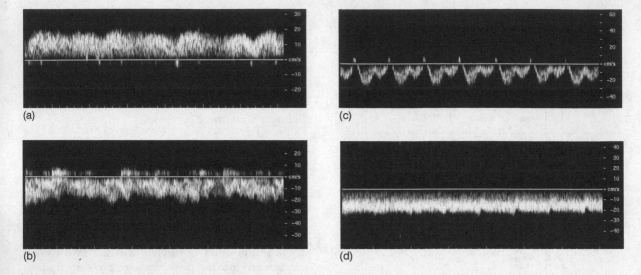

Figure 6.22 – Doppler waveforms obtained from the portal and hepatic veins. (a) Normal portal flow showing some pulsatility; (b) portal flow in a patient with cirrhosis (flow is reversed as hepatic arterial flow runs from the liver to portal collaterals); (c) normal hepatic vein showing pulsatile flow; (d) hepatic vein flow in a patient with cirrhosis (flow is continuous from a stiff liver).[11]

range of normal physiological control for maintaining cerebral blood flow at adequate levels (Figure 3.7).

Below the heart the increase in blood pressure leads to an increase in venous volume due to the large compliance of the veins. Valves in the veins prevent retrograde flow into this space but over the course of 1–2 min the veins fill from the arterial side until a complete fluid column is formed. As the valves reopen the full hydrostatic pressure then exists down the venous column of blood. Assuming there are no calf muscle contractions, by this stage, 500–600 ml blood has been transferred from the central venous circulation to the leg veins and a further 200–300 ml to the buttocks and pelvic area. If the legs are hot and the arterioles dilated, this filling can take place in a few seconds.

Because of the visco-elastic behaviour of vein walls there is a further increase in venous volume over time. This phenomenon is called **creep** as the walls stretch further under the increased pressure. The movement of blood into the venous space is known as **venous pooling**, which is a bit of a misnomer as blood still flows through the veins.

The increased transmural pressure at the capillary level also leads to leakage of plasma into the extravascular

Table 6.5 – Cardiovascular changes produced during a Valsalva manoeuvre

Increased intrathoracic and intra-abdominal pressure

Decreased venous return leading to reduced cardiac output

Response of increased heart rate and peripheral vasoconstriction

Decrease in transmural pressure in the aorta and all intrathoracic and intra-abdominal arteries

Reduction in pulse pressure and pulse wave velocity in aorta

Slow pulse wave velocity and short ventricular ejection greatly reduce reflected wave in aorta

Pulse pressure in upper limb is 1.5 times aortic pulse pressure (normally 0.5 times)

Amplification of the pressure wave between the central aorta and femoral artery tends to decrease

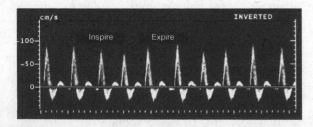

Figure 6.23 – Doppler waveform from the common femoral artery of a young, normal subject showing small changes in cardiac output with respiration.

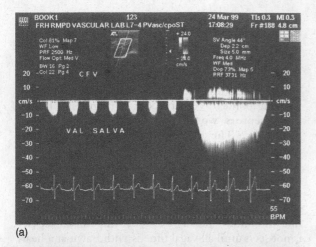

(a)

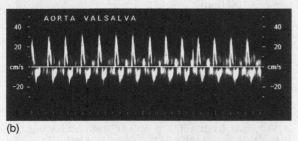

(b)

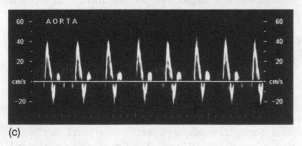

(c)

Figure 6.24 – Doppler waveforms showing the effects of a Valsalva manoeuvre on flow in (a) the common femoral vein and (b) the abdominal aorta. A normal aortic waveform is shown for comparison (c). Note the absence of phasic flow in the vein and tachycardia with low stroke volume in the artery.

fluid space and a 10% fall in plasma volume occurs fairly rapidly on standing. This leakage will eventually be self limiting as oncotic pressure rises to balance the hydrostatic pressure in the capillaries. However, if someone is placed in an upright tilt and supported so no weight is borne by the legs, then syncope will precede the equilibration of these pressures because the large reduction in central venous volume causes the cardiac output and blood pressure to fall. Maintenance of this position will eventually lead to death due to cerebral ischaemia. For a

body upright and submerged in water, the hydrostatic pressure of the water will counteract these effects since water has a similar density to blood.

The cardiovascular response to these changes brought on by an upright posture is to act to reverse their effect. Change in posture is sensed by the aortic and carotid sinus baroreceptors to produce the **aortic–carotid sinus baroreflex**. As the body moves into an upright position, the aortic receptors are lower than the carotid sinus receptors and the pressure difference between the two produces a signal proportional to sin θ, the angle of upright tilt.

The first response is a withdrawal of vagal tone to the heart. This occurs within one beat and leads to an immediate increase in heart rate. The increase in heart rate together with the drop in central venous volume means that the venous reservoir for the left ventricle is emptied within a few cardiac cycles. Stroke volume falls by 40% due to the operation of the Frank–Starling mechanism, and cardiac output decreases by 20% causing a further drop in arterial pressure. It takes 5–10 s for the sympathetic response to come into effect from the initial drop in carotid sinus pressure on standing. This produces vasoconstriction, especially in the hepatic–splanchnic region, the kidneys and the skin, so that blood is moved from these regions into the central veins, so restoring cardiac output (Figure 6.27).

When standing normally, even the small muscular contractions involved in maintaining an upright posture activate the calf muscle pump and aid venous return. Soldiers standing on parade are told to transfer their weight from one foot to the other and dorsiflex their toes to avoid fainting.

If orthostasis is prolonged the renin–angiotensin–aldosterone system is activated leading to water and sodium retention to increase plasma volume.

Orthostatic intolerance

Orthostatic intolerance resulting in **syncope**, or sudden loss of consciousness, may result from a number of causes. In every case syncope results from a precipitous decline in blood pressure and cerebral blood flow (CBF). If cerebral perfusion pressure falls < 50–60 mmHg, autoregulation fails and CBF falls. Below 40 mmHg there will be a loss of consciousness. Increasing cardiac output or increasing peripheral resistance can only increase arterial pressure. Unless venous return to the heart is increased, for example by vasoconstriction and activation of the calf muscle pump, cardiac output cannot be increased once central venous pressure falls to near zero (normal 5–8 mmHg).

Examples of orthostatic intolerance:

- It may occur **post-exercise** in runners who stand still after an exhaustive race so the calf muscle pump is stopped, the skin compartment is dilated, metabolic hyperaemia in muscle is high and venous return to the heart falls.

- During **heat stress**, total resistance drops causing central arterial pressure to fall by up to half the resting values as large flows are diverted to the skin. In the case of the skin there is no 'second heart' mechanism to aid venous return. Even activation of the calf muscle pump may not solve the problem because of the large proportion of blood not passing through the pump.

- So-called **vasovagal attack** occurs in some patients as a result of inappropriate vasodilatation together with profound bradycardia of vagal origin. This is due to a failure of the short-term mechanisms to maintain blood pressure. Bradycardia does not occur in all of these patients and peripheral vasodilatation alone can produce syncope. It is then referred to as **vasodepressor syncope**. In some patients with a hypersensitive carotid sinus reflex, a vasovagal attack may be clinically induced by **carotid sinus massage** in which the carotid baroreceptors are stimulated by manual pressure applied to the neck. This simulates the effect of high arterial pressure thereby increasing vagal outflow, decreasing sympathetic tone and prompting a vasovagal attack. The manifestation of this response is known as **carotid sinus syndrome**.

The placement of all these cases in a horizontal **recovery position** removes the displacement of blood by gravity so increasing ventricular filling, enabling CBF to be restored.

Exercise and conditioning

During exercise there is a large demand for oxygen from working skeletal muscle. This is met by vasodilatation producing a large increase in flow to the muscle. Mean blood pressure is maintained at close to normal levels during exercise indicating that the increase in cardiac output tending to increase blood pressure is matched by the drop in peripheral resistance of active muscle. The nature of the signals that initiate and maintain the close matching between blood flow and metabolism during exercise are still

not fully understood. Cardiovascular response to commencement of exercise is very rapid whereas reflexes from active muscle and its metabolic demands take time to build up. The immediate response appears to be due to withdrawal of vagal tone to the heart and resetting the baroreceptor reflex to a higher working point by cerebral control (Figure 6.11). The baroreceptors would then sense the pressure as hypotensive. The apparent deficit in pressure is then met first by an increase in heart rate due to vagal withdrawal and then by increasing sympathetic outflow (Figure 5.15). In a subject in whom stresses are applied at rest, sympathetic vasoconstriction is seen as soon as heart rate increases above a resting base line. In contrast, during exercise, sympathetic activity is not seen until all vagal tone is withdrawn at a heart rate of ~100 bpm.

Figure 6.25 shows the mechanisms involved in controlling blood pressure and flow during exercise and it illustrates the role of the venous reservoir.

As sympathetic activity increases, flow through the splanchnic region decreases linearly with increasing heart rate. The effect of this is to reduce splanchnic flow at $\dot{V}O_2$ *max* from 1500 to 350 ml min^{-1} allowing the redistribution of 1150 ml blood flow and 230 ml oxygen (1150 ml min^{-1} × 20 ml 100 ml^{-1}) to active muscle each minute. The splanchnic region itself survives by increasing its oxygen extraction from 4 to 17 ml 100 ml^{-1} blood (OER = 20–85%) after vasoconstriction. As severity of exercise increases, vasomotor control of active skeletal muscle becomes the most important target because only changes in its vascular conductance are then large enough to alter arterial pressure significantly. This begins at moderate exercise intensities, but blood flow remains high. When a large percentage of skeletal muscle is engaged in strenuous exercise, oxygen extraction (AVO$_2$ *diff*) by the muscle can equal that of the myocardium. When vigorous exercise is prolonged, body temperature increases and the highly compliant skin compartment vasodilates to move blood to the skin surface to effect cooling. The body then faces the greatest demand on the cardiovascular system, to supply both high demand from active muscles and the skin for cooling. The movement of blood volume to the skin inevitably produces a fall in ventricular filling pressure, and cardiac output can only be maintained by increasing heart rate, with increased oxygen extraction occurring in the tissue and increased oxygen uptake in the lungs. Figure 6.26 shows the changes in regional blood flow during exercise and Table 6.6 shows the changes in regional oxygen extraction accompanying the changes

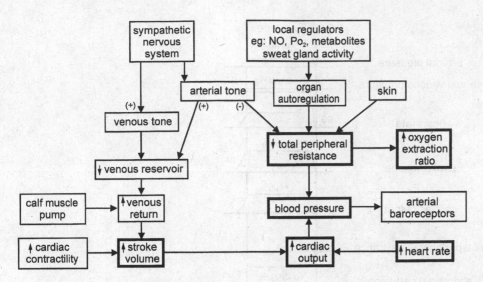

Figure 6.25 – Factors maintaining blood pressure during exercise including the role of the venous reservoir. At the commencement of exercise the arterial baroreceptors are reset at a higher level thereby triggering the events indicated.

in flow. Figure 6.27 shows the haemodynamic changes during exercise in comparison with those occurring following orthostasis.

Conditioning produced by a regular programme of exercise produces a 7–10% increase in total extraction

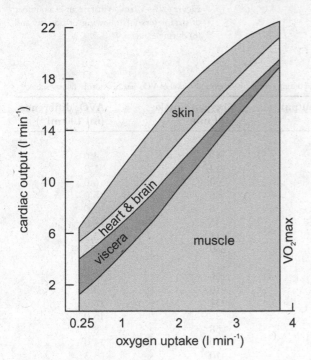

Figure 6.26 – Estimated distribution of cardiac output over the full range of oxygen uptake from rest to $\dot{V}O_2$ *max* at 3.7 l min^{-1}.[12]

of O_2. A greater percentage of cardiac output is directed to active muscle, which improves its conductance by removal of vasoconstrictor tone and increased capillary density. Reduction in resistance must be balanced by sufficient transit time to maximise O_2 extraction. The increase in muscle flow is provided by an increase in cardiac output sufficient to maintain blood pressure. A mild cardiac hypertrophy develops together with an improved O_2 supply to the myocardium. This reduces the wall tension required (Laplace equation) to meet the increase in volume load and stroke volume.

Effects of ageing

In describing the effects of ageing on the cardiovascular system we must distinguish between what are normal changes that occur throughout life and atherosclerosis which is a disease process and therefore an abnormality. Both processes produce detrimental effects that tend to manifest themselves after the age of 50. Atherosclerosis is particularly prevalent in populations in the developed world and so is frequently seen together with the normal ageing process seen in all populations. The effects of these two processes are quite different from each other (Table 6.7).

The most significant normal change with age is seen in the elastic walls of the central arteries of the body. This change increases the hydraulic load seen by the heart, which must then respond to maintain adequate circulation. The peripheral arteries change little with age and no change is seen in systemic or pulmonary veins.

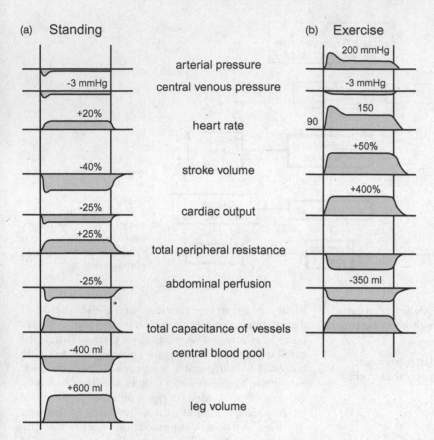

Figure 6.27 – Changes that occur in a number of parameters (a) following orthostasis and (b) during exercise.[14]

Table 6.6 – Estimated regional blood flow and oxygen consumption at rest (top) and during exercise (bottom) at the level of $\dot{V}O_2$ *max* in a normal human subject[4]

Region	Blood flow (ml min⁻¹)	Cardiac output (%)	Oxygen uptake (ml min⁻¹)	AVO₂ difference (ml 100 ml⁻¹)
At rest:				
Splanchnic	1500	27	60	4.0
Kidneys	1200	22	14	1.2
Muscle	1000(?)	18	60	6.0
Brain	750	14	60	8.0
Skin	500(?)	9	10	2.0
Coronary	250	5	35	14.0
Other	300(?)	5	11	3.7
Total	5500	100	250	4.5
During exercise:				
Splanchnic	350	1.4	60	17.0
Kidneys	360	1.4	10	3.6
Muscle (active)	21 800	87.4	3931	18.0
Muscle (inactive)	200	0.8	30	15.0
Brain	850	3.4	68	8.0
Skin	1000	4.0	140	14.0
Coronary	300	1.2	10	3.3
Other	100	0.4	11	11.0
Total	25 000	100.0	4260	17.0

Table 6.7 – Contrasting features of ageing change and atherosclerosis in human arteries[13]

	Atherosclerosis	Ageing change
Anatomic location	focal	diffuse in elastic arteries
Vascular location	intima	media
Vascular effect	constriction	dilatation
Consequence (distal)	ischaemia	nil
Consequence (proximal)	nil	LV load increased

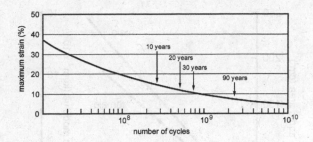

Figure 6.28 – Relationship between maximum strain ($\Delta l/l$) and number of cycles to fracture for natural rubber. Assuming elastin behaves like natural rubber, the number of cycles has been related to the age of an artery being cycled at average heart rate.[13]

Central elastic arteries

From 20 years of age, when the body is fully grown, changes occur in the arterial wall that are continuous and progressive throughout life. Intimal hyperplasia is seen even in the absence of atherosclerosis. Within the load-bearing medial layer there is a decrease in the number of elastin fibres and a change in their structure. The organised layers of elastin fibres gradually become frayed, with thinning and fragmentation of the fibres. With the degeneration of the elastin content, there is an increase in collagen fibres and a deposition of calcium which may be patchy or diffuse. These changes in the arterial wall cause the vessel to dilate and become tortuous.

The mechanism causing this degeneration of elastin in the media is probably mechanical fatigue due to repeated stressing of the fibres with pressure changes in each cardiac cycle. Turnover of elastin in arterial walls is very low with elastin fibres possibly lasting for life. The number of stress cycles they undergo is therefore extremely large.

Figure 6.28 shows the mean number of cycles before fracture for natural rubber. It depends on the percentage strain per cycle, which is given by:

Change in length/original length $\times$ 100 = % strain

Assuming that elastin behaves similarly to natural rubber, the mean time to fracture for several arterial percentage strains has been marked. This may be compared with Figure 6.29, which shows percentage strains measured in the carotid artery at various ages. A percentage strain of 10% is seen when < 30 years of age, falling to 5% at 70 years, indicating increasing

carotid stiffness. For comparison, peripheral arteries such as the radial artery have smaller strains of 2–4%. Based on the hypothesis of the mechanical fatigue of elastin, this is consistent with the peripheral arteries showing little disorganisation of elastin over a lifetime.

The result of these changes in wall structure with age are that the aorta increases in diameter, the elastic modulus increases so that the wall becomes stiffer and there is a decrease in the area ratio of the aortic bifurcation (A-I junction) so increasing the reflection coefficient (Figure 6.30).

The increase in elastic modulus produces an increase in the pulse wave velocity, the effect of increasing elastic modulus being greater than that of the increase in radius (see the Moens–Korteweg equation in Chapter 4).

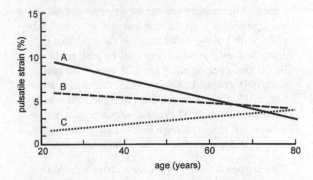

Figure 6.29 – Change in pulsatile strain (($D_S - D_D)/D_D$) with age for a normotensive carotid artery (A), a carotid artery in hypertensive subjects (B) and a radial artery in either (C). Note the decrease in carotid strain with age as the vessel becomes less elastic. In the hypertensive, the strain is less as the increased transmural pressure preloads the vessel. In the radial artery there is little change in elasticity with age but the pulse pressure in this vessel increases with age giving the increase in pulsatile strain shown (adapted from Boutouyrie *et al.* 1992).[15]

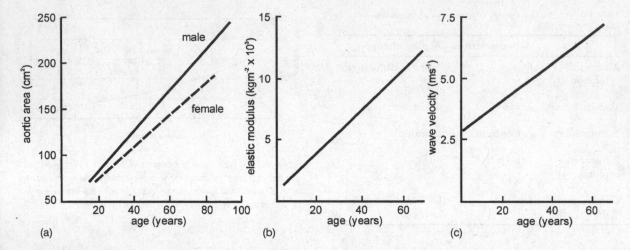

Figure 6.30 – Changes in the thoracic aorta with age showing change in (a) cross-sectional area,[16] (b) elastic modulus and (c) pulse wave velocity.[17]

This increase in pulse wave velocity in the aorta may be compared with a peripheral artery such as the brachial artery where pulse wave velocity is almost constant over four decades. This again indicates that the integrity of its wall structure does not change significantly with age.

Clinical note

Changes in Doppler waveforms with age

The Doppler waveforms seen in the neck and upper limb show the greatest change with age as a result of the reflected wave from the aortic bifurcation. The images shown in Figure 6.24 show three sets of images for comparison: a 9-year-old child with young elastic arteries, the length of the aorta was estimated by external measurement to be 30 cm; a young adult aged 25 years with aortic length 45 cm; and a 68-year-old male with aortic length 42 cm and no evidence of significant atherosclerotic disease. The child shows a much less prominent reflected wave on the descending slope of systole compared with the older man.

The shape of the Doppler waveforms seen in the common carotid artery is governed by the timing of the reflected wave from peripheral sites, effectively the aortic bifurcation, and the elasticity of the arteries themselves. As the aortic pulse wave velocity increases with age, the timing of the lower limb reflection moves from early diastole toward systole. The response of the carotid flow to this reflected wave depends on the elasticity of the carotid vessel wall, becoming smaller as the wall stiffens with age. In a young person, the reflected wave will cause a prominent dip in the descending slope of the systolic peak (Figure 6.31a) with elastic rebound of the carotid wall producing a noticeable second peak in the waveform. The dip from the reflected wave results from the fact that the flow wave is reflected in antiphase to the forward wave, as described in Chapter 4. In an older person with arteriosclerosis, the more prompt reflected wave and reduced wall elasticity produces a smaller dip in the descending systolic slope that is closer to peak systole. This typically gives a 'knee' appearance on the descending slope (Figure 6.31b). The dicrotic notch seen on young and old waveforms is produced by closure of the aortic valve at the end of systole.

The waveform seen in the ICA may come to resemble that seen in the CCA as arteriosclerosis progresses with age.

Impedance changes

Increasing pulse wave velocity and increasing mismatch in impedance at the aortic bifurcation changes the timing and amplitude of the reflected pulse wave in the aorta. This alters the input impedance seen by the heart. In the aorta, the pulse wave velocity more than doubles between 20 and 80 years giving a doubling of the characteristic impedance and a halving of the time for the reflected wave to return to the ascending aorta. The result is that the range of frequencies over which the impedance modulus is low, is narrowed and shifted to higher frequencies. In other words, there is a loss of the low impedance at low-frequency harmonics that is so advantageous to cardiac efficiency in young adults over the physiological range of heart rates (see Chapter 5). This is seen in the change in resting pulse pressure found in the ascending aorta. In young adults < 20 years of age, a pulse pressure of 25 mmHg is frequently seen; in octogenarians this can rise to 80 mmHg.

Figure 6.32 shows the effect of the progressive changes in ascending aortic impedance on the pressure and flow waves, together with the modulus of impedance spectra calculated from those waves.

Notes:

- The minima in the modulus of impedance shifts to higher frequencies with age. There is then a higher impedance at low harmonics giving a marked reduction in cardiac efficiency even by the age of 52.

- There is a gradual increase in characteristic impedance with age.

- There is an increase in pressure in late systole due to the reflected wave arriving back at the heart before systolic ejection is completed. This leads to a decreased ejection fraction from the heart during exercise.

- There is an early deceleration of aortic flow in late systole even in the absence of cardiac failure.

Clinical note
Brachial pressure measurements

Figure 6.33 shows the change in brachial and aortic pressure with age. For pressure measured in the brachial artery there is a rapid increase in systolic pressure during the adolescent years followed by a plateau from 20 to 50 years. During this period brachial systolic pressure is greater than that in the ascending aorta. This is due to amplification of the pulse pressure in the upper limb as a result of reflections from the lower limbs. In young adults the amplitude of the pressure pulse may be 50% greater in the brachial artery than in the ascending aorta. This is mainly seen in the systolic pressure, which

may be 20 mmHg higher. In the elderly the timing of the reflected component moves from early diastole to end-systole and the pulse pressure becomes the same as that in the ascending aorta, increasing with age after 50 years. Therefore, in terms of monitoring the deterioration of the vasculature with age, the brachial pressure plateau from 20 to 50 years of age may be considered an artefact that underestimates the continual increase in aortic pressure over this period.

Cardiac changes

Physical changes in the heart itself are relatively minor compared with those seen in the central elastic arteries. First there are cellular changes. No new cells are formed in the myocardium after neonatal development and there is then a gradual reduction in cell numbers and capillary density with age. The remaining cells tend to hypertrophy in response to increased ventricular workload so that ventricular wall thickness remains fairly constant, but nutrient perfusion is reduced. This hypertrophying is therefore a response to changes in the systemic arteries rather than changes in the heart *per se*. Second, there is some development of fibrous tissue producing a stiffening of the myocardium and a slower ventricular relaxation. This may lead to increased end-diastolic pressure and venous filling pressure, reducing the A-V pressure gradient in the coronary circulation and predisposing the myocardium to ischaemia. Third, there is a decrease in responsiveness to the sympathetic nervous system and circulatory hormones.

The increase in ventricular afterload moves the working point of the ventricular work cycle to the right, reducing coronary flow reserve (Figure 5.18b, curve C). Coronary flow reserve is further impaired by the changes in the aortic pressure wave brought about by changes in aortic impedance (Figure 6.34).

This shows two ascending aortic pressure waveforms, one typical of a more efficient arterial system seen in a young adult, the other produced by the early wave reflection seen in the elderly. This second waveform has a greater mean pressure difference between systole and diastole and diastolic pressure drops off rapidly. The effect of this is that the coronary artery has to supply oxygen for a greater ventricular afterload but with a reduced driving pressure in diastole. The A-V pressure

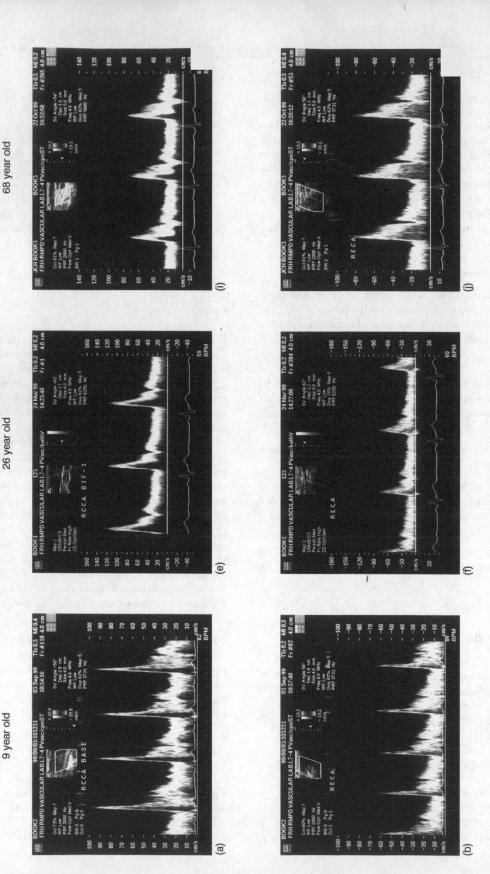

68 year old

26 year old

9 year old

148

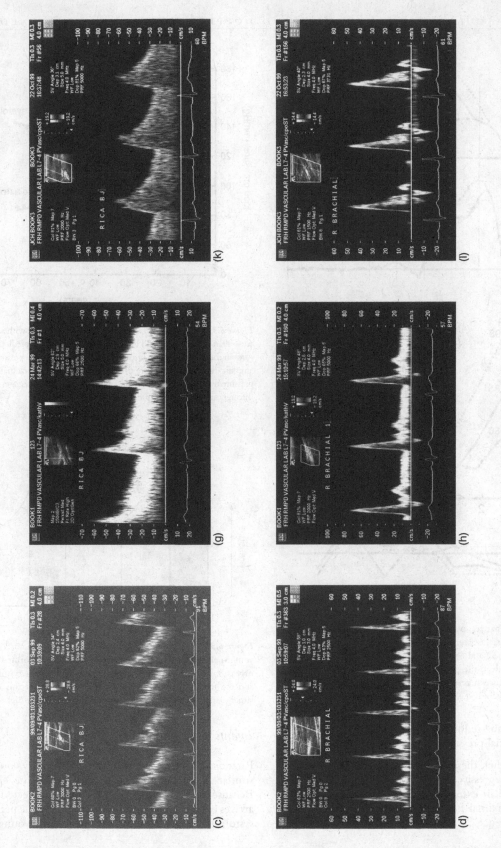

Figure 6.31 – Neck and upper limb waveforms for three subjects aged 9, 26 and 68 years.

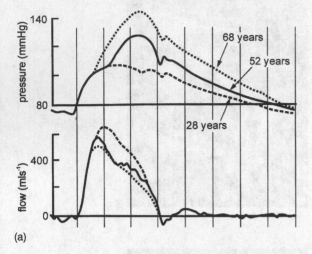

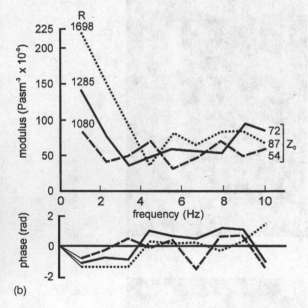

Figure 6.32 – Changes in pulse pressure waveform, flow waveform and impedance in the ascending aorta as seen in three normotensive subjects aged 28, 52 and 68 years. In (b) the impedance spectra have been calculated from the pressure and flow waves shown in (a). R, peripheral resistance at zero frequency; Z_0, characteristic impedance (adapted from Nichols *et al.* 1993).[18]

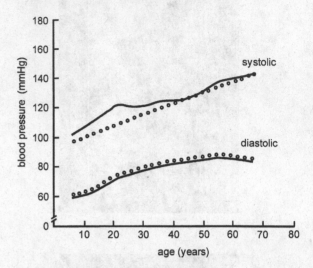

Figure 6.33 – Change in brachial arterial blood pressure with age in an Australian population (solid line). Dotted lines indicate predicted pressures in the aorta based on known differences in brachial pressure wave amplification with age. Note the plateau in measured brachial systolic pressure from 20 to 50 years whilst the aortic pressure increases linearly throughout adult life (adapted from ANHF 1989).[18,19]

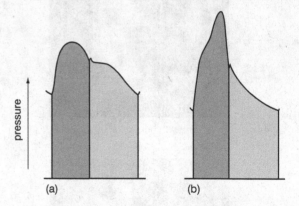

Figure 6.34 – Pressure waveforms from the proximal aorta in (a) a young person and (b) an elderly person. Work performed by the myocardium is proportional to the dark area under the systolic peak and the maximum systolic pressure. The oxygen for this work is largely supplied to the coronary arteries during diastole (light grey).[20]

gradient is thus reduced by both increased atrial and reduced arterial pressures.

Taken altogether, these changes in cardiac performance result in a progressive degradation in maximal exercise attainable and in extreme old age lead to heart failure. $\dot{V}O_2$ *max*, maximal heart rate, stroke volume, ejection fraction and hence cardiac output are all reduced with age.

Infants and children

Paradoxically, the waveforms seen in the very young are similar in appearance to those seen in the elderly. Because of their short body size, the reflected wave arrives back in the ascending aorta during the period of systole. Pulse wave velocity is typical of the young adult rather than the elderly, but the distance travelled is less. The length of systole is the same in children as it is in adults for any given heart rate and is not reduced in proportion to body size as might be expected.

Hypertension

Hypertension is a chronic and progressive increase in arterial blood pressure in which systolic pressure is > 140 mmHg (normal < 130 mmHg) and diastolic pressure is > 90 mmHg (normal < 85 mmHg). In 95% of cases there is no specific cause, when it is known as **essential hypertension**. Of the secondary causes, the two most common are renal parenchyma disease and renal artery stenosis.

Looking at the blood pressure equation (BP = CO × TVR), hypertension reflects a lack of control, producing too high a cardiac output, or too great a peripheral resistance, or inadequate renal excretion. This last factor is crucial for sustained hypertension to exist because the normal kidney is capable of reducing total fluid volume sufficiently to return blood pressure to normal.

In the early stages the elevated blood pressure is driven by increased cardiac output. In long-standing hypertensives cardiac output is normal or below normal and total peripheral resistance is chronically raised. The baroreflex still operates but is reset at a higher working point so that sympathetic tone is greater than normal. The haemodynamic effects are similar to the changes seen with ageing, only in the hypertensive they occur prematurely. Owing to pressure loading, the arterial wall compliance is decreased and it moves into the stiff collagen part of the compliance curve. This increases aortic impedance and pulse wave velocity giving an early-reflected wave. The arterial wall responds to these changes with intimal hyperplasia, smooth muscle hypertrophy, accelerated atherosclerosis and decreased endothelial function. Renin production is raised in 10% of cases or remains normal in 60% of cases. However, even normal production is too high in the hypertensive.

Every organ is affected, and the reduction in vessel calibre, the reduction in cardiac efficiency and inadequate renal excretion means that 'hypertension begets hypertension'. If left untreated, the condition is usually fatal. Of hypertensive patients, ~50% die of coronary artery disease or congestive heart failure, ~33% die from stroke and 10–15% from renal failure.

Arteriovenous fistula

An A–V fistula is often surgically created to allow access for dialysis in patients with end stage renal disease. These patients must be dialysed typically three times a week, with the dialyser requiring 300 ml min^{-1} to run. It is not possible to access an artery repeatedly because of the problems associated with the arterial wall fibrosing and thrombosis. Neither is it possible to draw 300 ml min^{-1} from a vein as the pressure is not sufficient and the vein will just collapse. By creating a fistula, an arterial flow is created in a vein that can be repeatedly accessed. However, such a fistula is the equivalent of a short circuit in the cardiovascular circulation. The resistance to flow is very low and as much as 2–2.5 l min^{-1} may go from the heart to the fistula and straight back to the heart, imposing a large volume workload on the heart even at rest. The fact that fistulas are so well tolerated by the heart shows that the heart is better able to cope with an increase in volume load compared with an increased pressure load, which is deleterious if not corrected.

An example of flow to an A–V fistula is shown in Figure 6.35. Note the high velocities seen throughout the cardiac cycle. The measurement was made in the brachial artery supplying the fistula. A straight segment of artery was aligned with the ultrasound probe and the sample volume set to straddle the vessel. Time-averaged velocity was measured over a complete number of cardiac cycles and the vessel diameter carefully measured. TAV = 31.2 cm^{-1}, cross-sectional area = 0.34 cm^2, giving a volume flow of 636 ml min^{-1}. Reynolds number Re = 542 and the flow, although high, is not turbulent.

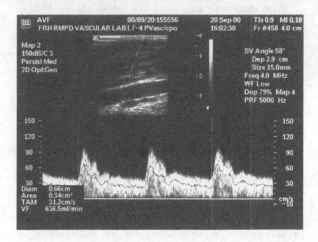

Figure 6.35 – Doppler waveform with measurements obtained from the brachial artery of a patient with an arteriovenous fistula in the radial artery surgically created for haemodialysis access.

Diabetes

Diabetes affects both the microvascular circulation, for example producing retinopathy and affecting kidney function, and the major arteries. Coronary artery disease is more common in these patients with an increased risk of mortality rate following a myocardial infarction. They are also at greater risk of stroke. Mild hypertension (135–140 mmHg systolic pressure) is often seen associated with nephropathy.

Disease in the lower limb arteries is a common vascular complication in diabetics. Compared with non-diabetics, it tends to be bilateral and more extensive and with narrowing particularly prevalent in the distal tibial vessels. This affects flow to the foot, which together with small vessel disease and neuropathy produces the 'diabetic foot'. When there is vascular involvement, ischaemic lesions of the foot may be seen.

Clinical note
Doppler measurements in diabetics

A common observation in scanning diabetic patients is a good-calibre lumen throughout the lower limb but with extensive calcification in the medial layer of the arteries. This makes the arterial wall more rigid and has the effect of increasing the pulse wave velocity and producing a Doppler waveform with a very fast rise time (SRT < 60 ms). Whilst flow may remain pulsatile to ankle level, volume flow is quite poor as the distal vessels tend to be narrow. Ankle pressure measurements are falsely elevated due to the rigidity of the vessel wall. It is often difficult to determine accurately the exact point at which flow is cut off and recommences as the pressure cuff is inflated and deflated. When this occurs or the pressures measured are very high, caution must be exercised when interpreting the results.

Cerebral circulation

The brain can safeguard its own oxygen supply by controlling cardiac output and the vascular resistance of other organs. **Cerebral blood flow** (CBF) is strongly regulated by autoregulation of the pressure–flow relationship and by responding to changes in blood gases. With the exception of the heart, perfusion of other organs may be sacrificed to preserve cerebral perfusion when necessary. There is

also strong localised control related to tissue metabolism within the brain itself.

The grey matter of the brain has a very high metabolic rate so that it takes 14% of resting cardiac output and uses 3–3.5 ml $100g^{-1}$ min^{-1} arterial oxygen or 15–20% total resting oxygen consumption. Total cerebral blood flow is ~750 ml min^{-1}. Over the autoregulatory range blood flow falls by ~45 ml min^{-1} for every 10 mmHg drop in **cerebral perfusion pressure** (CPP). When CPP falls below 50 mmHg cerebral autoregulation fails and CBF becomes dependent on pressure, with the drop in flow resulting in mental confusion and syncope. Consciousness is lost within a few seconds of ischaemia with irreversible cell damage occurring after ~4 min. This period is prolonged when there is hypothermia. In terms of flow, clinical symptoms appear if the flow falls below ~560 ml min^{-1} and syncope is likely when flow falls to < 390 ml min^{-1}.

Flow to the brain is through the carotid and vertebral arteries with the majority of flow passing via the internal carotid arteries. The main baroreceptor is in the carotid sinus so cerebral arterial pressure is directly monitored. The arteries pass into the skull, which forms a rigid box of fixed volume. The vertebral arteries join to form the basilar artery, which is connected by a set of small communicating vessels with the carotid arteries to form the Circle of Willis. This provides a degree of protection in the event of reduction of flow in one of the main supplying arteries as collateral flow can pass from one side to the other. Flow in these small communicating vessels is usually low as pressures are balanced on each side.

Clinical note
Superficial temporal artery compression test

When there is severe disease in the internal carotid artery, a significant proportion of cerebral flow may be supplied via the collateral route of the external carotid–superficial temporal–orbital–ophthalmic artery. The degree to which this route is active can be assessed by examining flow in the supra-orbital and supertrochlear arteries that connect the extra-to the intracranial arteries through the orbit.

In a normal subject the internal carotid artery is a low-resistance path and the external carotid artery is a high-resistance path. With these two paths forming parallel resistances (Figures 3.11 and 3.29), flow will normally be out of the orbit as this is the path of least resistance. When ICA resistance is increased by disease, flow into the orbit becomes the path of least resistance. The effect of these changes can be demonstrated by manually compressing the superficial temporal artery against the bone whilst simultaneously observing flow in either of the orbital arteries (Figure 6.36). Table 6.8 and Figure 6.37 show the results for this test.

Table 6.8 – Diagnostic criteria for the ophthalmic artery compression test

	Normal	Severe ICA disease
STA uncompressed	flow out of orbit	flow into orbit
STA compressed	flow out of orbit enhanced	flow ceases or is reversed

Normally carotid flow supplies the anterior and lateral parts of the cerebral cortex, and the vertebral arteries supply the posterior circulation including the cerebellum, pons and medulla. Hypotension in the posterior circulation produces vertigo, for example where vertebral arteries are diseased. **Postural hypotension** is produced in orthostasis through a reduction in hydrostatic pressure. Control of CBF is at the level of the

smaller arteries and arterioles, which have richly innervated smooth muscle walls. Capillary density is high and the capillaries are isolated from cerebral interstitial fluid by tight junctions between the capillary endothelial cells. This forms what is known as the **blood–brain barrier** that prevents many water-soluble and large molecular weight substances from passing into the brain. Venous drainage is via large venous sinuses that run superficially over the brain and drain mainly via the internal jugular vein and also by channels which run to the vertebral and peri-orbital veins.

Blood flow to the brain is complicated by two factors. First, the skull forms a rigid box of fixed volume. Second, with an upright posture, there is a negative hydrostatic pressure in the skull relative to the right atrium of the heart.

Within the skull there are effectively three compartments occupying the space: the brain mass (80%), the blood (10%) and cerebrospinal fluid (10%). **Cerebrospinal fluid** (CSF) is found in the subarachnoid space where it bathes the brain and extends down to the base of the spinal cord forming a continuous column of fluid. CSF is continually produced at 0.5 ml min^{-1} from secretory epithelial cells in the choroid plexus, which is well supplied by a capillary network, and is reabsorbed back into the venous sinuses within the cranium. Total volume of CSF is 120 ml. Because the volume of the skull is fixed,

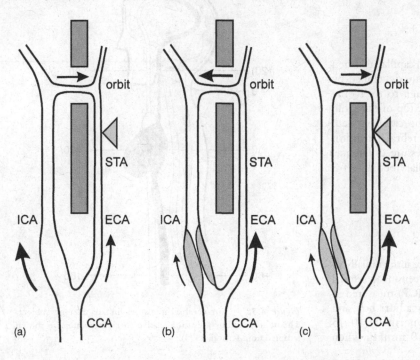

Figure 6.36 – Superficial temporal artery (STA) compression test for orbital flow. Arrows indicate the relative size and direction of flow: (a) normal situation with flow out of orbit via the internal carotid artery (ICA); (b) severe ICA disease with flow into the orbit via the external carotid artery; (c) when STA-compressed flow into the orbit is reversed.

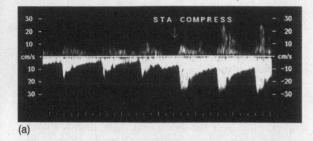

(a)

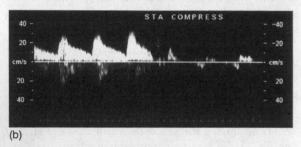

(b)

Figure 6.37 – Doppler waveforms obtained from the supra-orbital artery during the superficial temporal artery compression test: (a) normal response, flow out of the orbit is enhanced upon compression of the superficial temporal artery; (b) flow into the orbit is abolished upon compression in a patient with bilateral ICA occlusion.

the volume V of each compartment can only expand with a reciprocal decrease of another:

$$V_{\text{cranial contents}} = V_{\text{brain}} + V_{\text{blood}} + V_{\text{CSF}}$$

For blood to flow through the cerebral capillaries when a person is standing, the blood pressure developed by the left ventricle must be great enough to overcome the drop in hydrostatic pressure to the top of the skull, and the resistance to perfusion of the capillary bed. Cerebral blood flow depends on cerebral perfusion pressure (CPP), which is the A-V pressure difference, and the vascular resistance of the capillary bed:

$$\text{CBF} = \frac{\text{CPP}}{R_{\text{vasc}}}$$

Cerebral Blood Flow

It is not easy to measure venous pressure intracranially so CPP is taken to be the difference between mean arterial pressure and **intracranial pressure** (ICP) measured in CSF. ICP may be measured by making a burr hole and inserting a pressure transducer. It is normally 10–15 mmHg when lying supine and 5–10 mmHg when

upright. This drop with change in posture is the change in hydrostatic pressure. Because the CSF is external to the blood space it has the effect of ameliorating the fall in cerebral perfusion pressure that results from the drop in hydrostatic pressure in the arterial supply. That is, the low CSF pressure is potentially able to increase the transmural pressure in capillaries and veins within the skull and help keep them open. This is the opposite of the phenomenon where blood is pushed back to the heart when an upright subject is submersed in water. There the hydrostatic pressure of the water balances the increase in hydrostatic pressure in the lower limbs. With the top of the skull some 400 mm above the heart the mean arterial pressure is 60 mmHg implying a cerebral perfusion pressure of $\geq$ 50–60 mmHg throughout the brain (Figure 6.38).

Within the skull the venous pressure is negative with respect to the heart, but the veins are kept partially open by their tethering to adjacent structures. However, the jugular vein collapses when it passes outside the skull so there is not a continuous fluid column or siphon extending from the heart to inside the head.

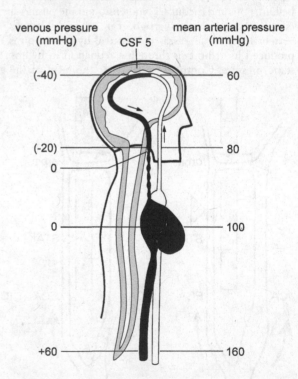

Figure 6.38 – Intracerebral pressures in an upright subject. Theoretical venous pressures relative to right atrium are shown (adapted from Rowell 1993).[12]

As the size of the brain is normally constant, change in cerebral blood volume must be counterbalanced by movement of CSF out of the skull. Within the brain there are large regional changes in blood flow that vary with mental activity and local metabolic control. Sympathetic vasomotor control in the brain appears to be very small in humans with no response to even powerful baroreflexes.

Cerebral blood flow has a very high response to variations in blood gases. In particular, it responds to changes in PCO_2 (Figure 6.39a). Inhalation of 5% CO_2 producing an excess of CO_2 known as **hypercapnia** will lead to a 50% increase in cerebral blood flow. The sensitivity to PO_2 is low until it falls to < 50 mmHg (Figure 6.39b). Inhalation of 7% O_2 producing an

oxygen deficit or **hypoxaemia** will produce a 100% increase in cerebral blood flow.

As oxygen saturation of arterial blood is almost complete at normal oxygen pressure and ventilation rate, voluntary hyperventilation has the effect of driving off more CO_2 leading to **hypocapnia**. The vasoconstriction resulting from this washout of CO_2 can reduce CBF by as much as 35%. This is sufficient to cause cerebral ischaemia with symptoms of dizziness and tingling. However, during hypoxaemia, for example when O_2 demand is high, reflex hyperventilation still reduces arterial PCO_2. The vasoconstrictor effects of hypocapnia then compete with the vasodilator effects of hypoxia and cerebral blood flow tends to fall during severe exercise. These mechanisms are also important during exposure to high altitude and when a person suffers from anaemia.

Following a haemorrhagic stroke, trauma to the head or the growth of a tumour, the intracranial volume of CSF is reduced by its movement outside the skull and by increased absorption reducing its total volume. If there is an over production of CSF or when these compensatory mechanisms are exhausted, ICP will rise. In the case of stroke or trauma, a rapidly expanding mass such as a haematoma or inflammation produces an immediate rise in ICP. This acts to compress the small vessels and capillaries in the manner of a Starling resistor. This then prompts a strong response of generalised peripheral vasoconstriction in the body, and reflex bradycardia that raises blood pressure to maintain cerebral perfusion, known as the **Cushing reflex**. It can restore and maintain CBF in the short term, but the increased cardiac afterload can lead to elevated left atrial and pulmonary arterial pressures so that pulmonary oedema results. In the case of cerebral haemorrhage, the increase in pressure often results in further bleeding into CSF, which in turn makes CBF fall further – a positive feedback loop. A second detrimental mechanism that may occur in the brain-damaged patient is the failure of autoregulation so that blood flow passively follows pressure changes. If CPP then rises to > 150 mmHg as a result of the Cushing reflex, the resultant disruption of the blood–brain barrier leads to cerebral oedema, further increasing ICP. This process is known as **vasodilatory cascade** and can be difficult to control with fatal consequences.

Pulmonary circulation

The pulmonary circulation is a low-pressure circulation through which almost the entire cardiac output passes. Systolic pressure in the normal pulmonary artery is

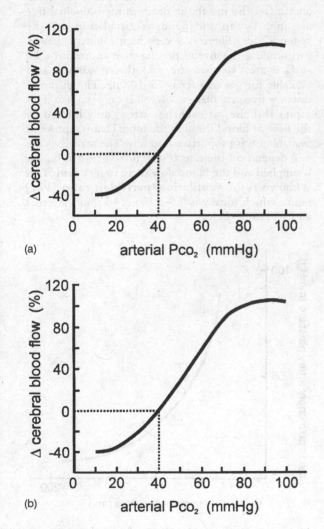

Figure 6.39 – Response of cerebral blood flow to (a) changes in arterial PCO_2 and (b) arterial PO_2.

15–25 mmHg and diastolic pressure is 8–15 mmHg. Total resistance to flow is only one-sixth that of the systemic circulation and with little muscle in the short arterioles, resistance is more evenly distributed across the circuit than for systemic vessels. There is no autoregulation of flow in the lungs. Resistance is 30% arterial, 50% arterioles to venules and 20% venous. The mean capillary pressure of 8–11 mmHg therefore lies about half way between the mean arterial (12–15 mmHg) and venous (5–8 mmHg) pressures. Although the pulse pressure is lower than on the systemic side, the distribution of resistance means that some 5–10% of the pulsation is transmitted through to the pulmonary veins. In the pulmonary arteries the acceleration in systole is slower so the waveforms have a more rounded appearance and the waveform shape of the pressure and flow waves are similar (Figure 6.40).

This is because the global reflection coefficient for the pulmonary arterial tree is low. The modulus of impedance shows a similar pattern to that seen in the aorta with a minimum value occurring for the low harmonic components of the pulse waveforms. In the pulmonary arterial tree the short distance to the site of reflection is matched by a slower pulse wave velocity of ~2.5 ms⁻¹, so the reflected wave arrives back at the pulmonary valve in a similar time to that arriving back at the aortic valve.

There is no change in impedance with normal breathing, but pulmonary hypertension does produce a change. **Pulmonary hypertension** may be caused by heart failure, mitral valve regurgitation or pulmonary disease raising pulmonary resistance. The impedance then increases as the vascular compliance decreases and the waveforms

look more like aortic waveforms with a fast systolic rise time. Figure 6.41 shows how the systolic rise time in the pulmonary artery is related to the pulmonary arterial pressure, and may be used as a measure of it.

This change in vascular impedance makes the coupling of the right ventricle to pulmonary artery less efficient and so increases the work demand on the heart. In addition, a pulmonary vein pressure of 20–25 mmHg raises capillary pressure sufficiently to cause pulmonary oedema. Oedema reduces gas exchange and makes the lungs less compliant and therefore more difficult to inflate. Breathing becomes difficult and uncomfortable – a condition known as **dyspnoea**.

Pulmonary blood flow far exceeds nutritional needs and in fact the metabolic needs of the bronchial tree are met by an independent circulation on the systemic side. There is a very high capillary density surrounding the alveoli that have an enormous total surface area so that the endothelial surface area available for gas transfer is 75–100 m². The diffusion distance from capillary to alveoli is only 0.3 μm. This means that the gas exchange rate is only limited by the flow of blood through the lung. That is, uptake of available O_2 is proportional to flow. The actual uptake will depend on the rate at which oxygen-bearing air is supplied and the blood flow there to pick it up. This is known as the **ventilation/perfusion ratio** ($\dot{V}/\dot{Q}$ ratio), which ideally is 0.8–1.0, i.e. 4 l min⁻¹ alveolar air to 5 l min⁻¹ blood.

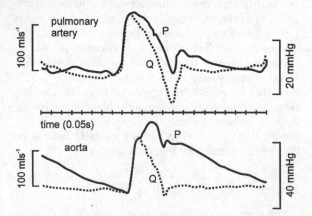

Figure 6.40 – Pulse pressure (P) and flow (Q) waveforms for pulmonary artery and ascending aorta in a dog.[21]

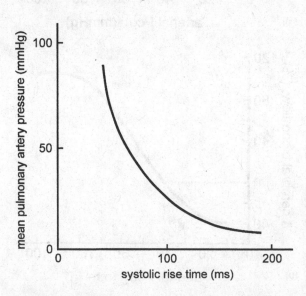

Figure 6.41 – Relationship between increasing pulmonary artery pressure and systolic rise time in the pulmonary artery.[12]

In the lung of an upright person there is a gradient of hydrostatic pressure. This causes the capillaries and veins at the apex of the lung to collapse during diastole and the vessels below the level of the heart to become distended (Figure 6.42). There is therefore a higher $\dot{V}/\dot{Q}$ ratio at the apex than at the base, and the efficiency of blood oxygenation in a resting upright person is lower than when they are supine. The diffusion capacity of the lung is increased by up to 20% when lying down because the blood supply is more evenly distributed in the lung and pulmonary blood volume increases.

If ventilation to a local region of lung falls or local blood flow increases, then the alveolar PO_2 will decrease and PCO_2 will increase. This causes small pulmonary arteries that pass close to the surface of small airways to respond to the hypoxia by vasoconstricting so reducing blood flow. The bronchiolar smooth muscle responds to the airway hypercapnia by relaxing. These two responses ensure that the $\dot{V}/\dot{Q}$ ratio is maintained close to the ideal. Notice that the arterial response of vasoconstriction to hypoxia is the opposite of that which occurs in systemic ischaemia when vasodilatation occurs. This mechanism ensures that blood flow is always directed towards the well-oxygenated regions of the lung, which in some diseases becomes patchy. The rate and depth of inspiration is such as to minimise the work done by the respiratory muscles in providing adequate ventilation whether at rest or during exercise.

During physical exercise in an upright subject a modest rise in pulmonary artery pressure allows the vessels in the apex to open up and thereby increase gas exchange. This process of bringing more vessels into active service is known as **recruitment**. During exercise the oxygen transfer capability of the lung can increase by 70%. This results from increased alveolar ventilation and an increase in capillary blood volume from 85 to 180 ml leading to an improved diffusion area and $\dot{V}/\dot{Q}$ ratio.

Total blood volume in the lungs of a supine subject is 600 ml, but due to the high distensibility of the circuit this may vary between 300 ml upon performing a Valsalva manoeuvre to 1000 ml upon performing a Müller manoeuvre. The capacitance of the lung acts as a transient source of blood for the left ventricle when cardiac output is increased.

Complete cardiovascular system

We are now in a position to have an overview of the whole cardiovascular system in terms of its functionality and control (Figure 6.43). This diagram is a synthesis of all the system diagrams used in this chapter and in Chapter 5. The key parameters that must be regulated are shown in bold boxes. The arrows show the direction of action.

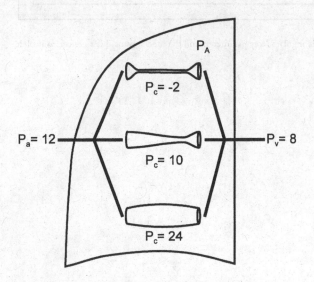

Figure 6.42 – Variation in perfusion in the lung of an upright subject.

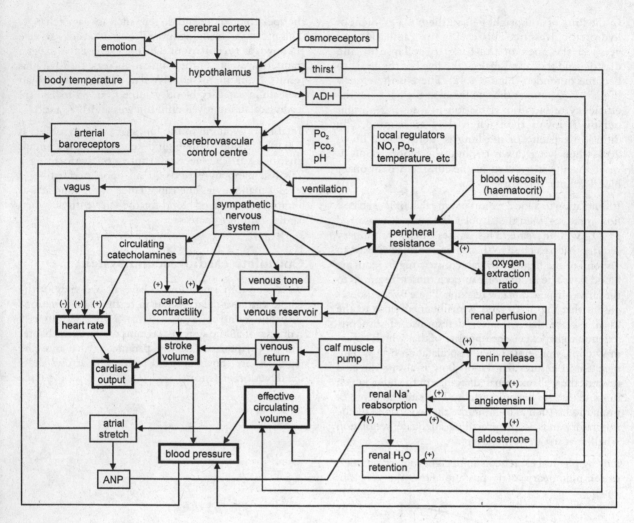

Figure 6.43 – Overview of the whole cardiovascular system in terms of the regulated key parameters and the mechanisms able to effect control. It is a synthesis of Figures 5.6, 6.7, 6.16 and 6.25.

References

1. Harkness MLR, Harkness RD, McDonald DA. The collagen and elastin content of the arterial wall in the dog. *Proceedings of the Royal Society of London* 1957; **164B**: 541–551.

2. Lilly LS (ed.). *Pathophysiology of Heart Disease*. Baltimore: Williams & Wilkins, 1998.

3. Milnor WR. *Hemodynamics*. Baltimore: Williams & Wilkins, 1982.

4. Rowell LB. *Human Cardiovascular Control*. Oxford: Oxford University Press, 1993.

5. Landgren S. *Acta Physiologica Scandinavica* (1952) **26**: 35–56. The baroreceptor activity in the carotid sinus nerve and the distensibility of the sinus wall.

6. Celander O. *Acta Physiologica Scandinavica* (1954) **32 (suppl. 116)**: 1–132. The range of control exercised by the sympathetico-adrenal system.

7. Little RC, Little WC. *Physiology of the Heart and Circulation*, 4th edn. Chicago: Year Book, 1989.

8. Berne RM, Levy MN. *Cardiovascular Physiology*, 3rd edn. St Louis: CV Mosby, 1977.

9. Levick JR. *An Introduction to Cardiovascular Physiology*. Oxford: Butterworth-Heinemann, 1995.

10. Rowell B (1983) Cardiovascular adjustments to thermal Stress. In: Shepherd JT, Abboud FM and Geiger SR (eds) Handbook of Physiology. The cardiovascular system: Peripheral circulation and organ blood flow sect 2, vol III part 2 p967–1023.

11. Bolondi L, Bassi SL, Gaiani S *et al*. Liver cirrhosis: changes of Doppler waveform of hepatic veins. *Radiology* 1991; **178**: 513–516.

12. Rowell LB. *Human Cardiovascular Control*. Oxford: Oxford University Press, 1993.

13. Nichols WW, O'Rourke MF. *Mcdonald's Blood Flow in Arteries*, 4th edn. London: Arnold, 1998.

14. Schmidt RF, Thews G. *Human Physiology*. Berlin: Springer, 1983.

15. Boutouyrie P, Laurent S, Bentos A *et al*. Opposing effects of aging on distal and proximal large arteries in hypertensives. *Journal of Hypertension* 1992; **10 (suppl. 6)**: 591–597.

16. Mitchell JRA, Schwartz CJ. *Arterial Disease*. Philadelphia: FA Davis, 1965.

17. Gozna ER, Marble AE, Shaw A, Holland JG. Age-related changes in the mechanics of the aorta and pulmonary artery of man. *Journal of Applied Physiology* 1974; **36**: 407–411.

18. Nichols WW, Avolio AP, Kelly RP *et al*. Effects of age and of hypertension on wave travel and reflections. In MF O'Rourke, M Safae, V Dzau (eds) *Arterial Vasodilation: Mechanisms and Therapy*. London: Edward Arnold, 1993: 23–40.

19. Preliminary survey analysis in Risk Factor Prevalence Study, In: Risk Factor Prevalence Study (ed) Survey No3 (1989), Australian National Heart Foundation: Canberra.

20. O'Rourke MF. *Arterial Function in Health and Disease*. Edinburgh: Churchill Livingstone, 1982.

21. Van den Bos GC, Westerhof N, Randall OS. Pulse wave reflection: can it explain the differences between systemic and pulmonary pressure and flow waves? *Circulation Research* 1982; **51**: 479–485.

22. Kitabatake A, Inoue M, Masuyama T *et al*. Noninvasive evaluation of pulmonary hypertension by a pulsed Doppler technique. *Circulation* 1983; **68**: 302–309.

Further reading

Folkow B, Svanborg A. Physiology of cardiovascular aging. *Physiological Reviews* 1993; **73**: 725–764.

Lote CJ. *Principles of Renal Physiology*, 3rd edn. London: Chapman & Hall, 1994.

Matthews LR. *Cardiopulmonary Anatomy and Physiology*. Philadelphia: Lippincott, 1996.

Moreno AH, Burchell AR. Respiratory regulation of splanchnic and systemic venous return in normal subjects and in patients with hepatic cirrhosis. *Surgery, Gynaecology and Obstetrics* 1982; **154**: 257–267.

Nichols WW, O'Rourke MF. *Mcdonald's Blood Flow in Arteries*, 4th edn. London: Arnold, 1998.

Quan KJ, Carlson MD, Thames MD. Mechanisms of heart rate and arterial blood pressure control: Implications for the pathophysiology of neurocardiogenic syncope. *Pacing and Clinical Electrophysiology* 1997; **20**: 764–774.

Reid IA. Interactions between ANGII, sympathetic nervous system, and baroreceptor reflexes in regulation of blood pressure. *American Journal of Physiology* 1992; **262**: E763–778.

Sagnella GA, MacGregor GA. Atrial natriuretic peptides. *Quarterly Journal of Medicine*, n.s. 77, 1990; **282**: 1001–1007.

Seymour RS. Model analogues in the study of cephalic circulation. *Comparative Biochemistry and Physiology Part A* 2000; **125**: 517–524.

APPENDICES

APPENDIX A:
THE WINDKESSEL MODEL

Historically, the coupling between the heart and the systemic vasculature has been modelled by considering the arterial tree to be a compliant elastic chamber with an outflow presenting a fluid resistance. The ventricle is then an intermittent pump ejecting its stroke volume into this compliant chamber. This model of the cardiovascular system is known as the windkessel model after the old German fire engines that had an air-filled compression chamber, or windkessel, fitted between the water pump and the outflow hose (Figure A.1a). The effect of the windkessel was to smooth out any oscillations in the pumped water so a continuous jet of water left the hose. By analogy, the compliance of the major arteries smooths out the intermittent flow of the heart to give a continuous blood supply to the peripheral vascular bed.

The windkessel model is a **lumped parameter model** in that all the variation that occurs along the length of the arterial tree is summed up in a single capacitance and resistance (Figure A.1b). For this reason, the model cannot take into account many of the features of pulsatile flow seen in real arteries. In particular, it cannot account for wave propagation phenomena, including reflections, that occur as a result of the pulse wave having a finite velocity along a branching tube whose impedance changes from point to point.

Where the windkessel model has been useful is in modelling ventricular–vascular coupling from the point of view of the ventricle. This is because it treats the ventricle and the vascular properties as independent of one another, which to a large extent is true since vessel impedance depends only on the properties of the vessel itself, not the shape of the pulse wave entering it. Using a windkessel model has enabled pressure–volume relationships within the left ventricle to be studied and has produced predictions and values that closely match real values measured *in vivo*. The model, used in dogs, successfully predicted stroke volume, stroke work, oxygen consumption, and systolic and diastolic aortic pressures reasonably close to those found when true impedance was used. However, it could not accurately predict the pressure and flow waveforms since these depend on the timing of forward and reflected pulses. The ventricular pressure–volume diagrams used in Chapter 5 are based on a three-element windkessel model.

Reference

1. O'Rourke MF. *Arterial Function in Health and Disease.* Edinburgh: Churchill Livingstone, 1982.

Further reading

Kass DA, Kelly RP. Ventriculo-arterial coupling: concepts, assumptions and applications. *Annals of Biomedical Engineering* 1992; **20**: 41–62.

Nichols WW, O'Rourke MF. *Mcdonald's Blood Flow in Arteries*, 4th edn. London: Arnold, 1998.

Sunagawa K, Maughan L, Burkhoff D, Sawagwa K. Left ventricular interaction with arterial load studied in isolated canine ventricle. *American Journal of Physiology* 1983; **245**: H733–780.

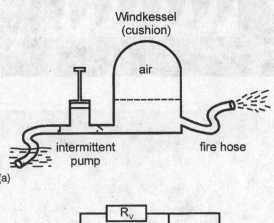

(a)

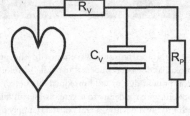

(b)

Figure A.1 – (a) Windkessel fire pump; (b) equivalent electrical circuit when modelling the cardiovascular system. C_v, vascular capacitance; R_v, proximal vascular resistance; R_p, peripheral resistance.[1]

APPENDIX B: HAEMODYNAMICS APPLIED

This Appendix presents further examples of Doppler waveforms and shows how the physical principles discussed in other chapters apply in practice. The descriptions illustrate the sort of thought processes that should go on in the mind of the operator performing the scan as they arrive at a reasoned conclusion for the report they must write at the end.

Proximal disease progression

Figure B.1 shows a sequence of waveforms that indicates progression of proximal arterial disease. In this case, the waveforms are taken from the common femoral artery (CFA) and indicate worsening aorto-iliac disease.

1   Shows the normal triphasic waveform. There is a fast systolic rise time (SRT; 90 ms) with a window under the systolic peak indicating plug flow in a smooth vessel.

(2, 3) When there is mild aorto-iliac disease there is a loss of the third component and the systolic window may begin to fill due to disturbed flow transmitted downstream from an uneven lumen. As the disease progresses the systolic peak broadens and there is a gradual loss of the second component of the waveform. SRT time is still fairly rapid.

4   When there is severe disease or a proximal occlusion, so flow to the CFA is via collaterals, the waveform is fully damped. Now SRT >130 ms (245 ms here) and there is forward flow throughout the cardiac cycle.

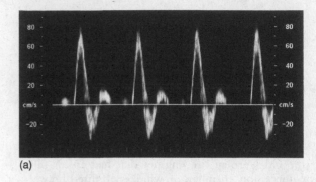

(a)

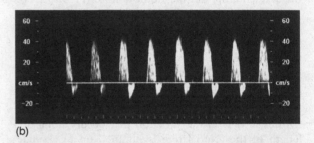

(b)

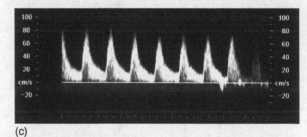

(c)

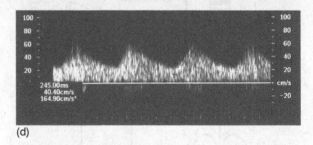

(d)

Figure B.1 – Common femoral waveforms in the presence of progressing proximal disease: (a) normal triphasic waveform; (b) loss of the third component due to mild proximal disease; (c) loss of the second component with moderate to severe disease; (d) fully damped waveform with proximal occlusion and collateral supply to CFA.

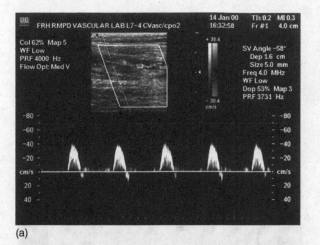

(a)

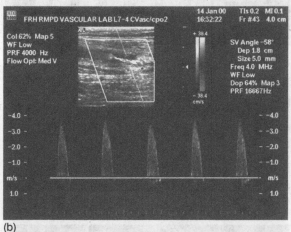

(b)

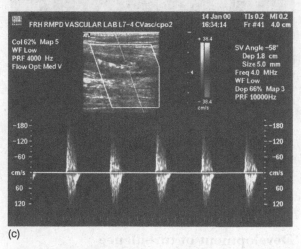

(c)

Figure B.2 – Change in flow through a stenosis: (a) pulsatile waveform proximal to the stenosis; (b) very high velocities within the tight stenosis; (c) turbulent flow as fast jet runs into wide vessel distal to the stenosis.

Change in flow through a stenosis

Figure B.2 shows the changes in waveform seen in a typical SFA stenosis. Figure B.2a shows pulsatile flow immediately proximal to the stenosis. There is a window under the systolic peak indicating laminar plug flow, although the velocities are somewhat lower than normal because of the resistance to flow presented by the stenosis. Within the stenosis itself, Figure B.2b shows very high peak systolic velocities of 3.8 ms^{-1} occurring as the vessel cross-sectional area is greatly reduced. Figure B.2c shows post-stenotic turbulence where the fast jet enters a wider vessel lumen so the Reynolds number is large. Within the turbulent flow, complex streamline paths exist with flow occurring in both directions at once within the sample volume, which has been set to straddle the vessel.

Subclavian steal

The pressures in each vertebral artery are normally the same and equal that in the proximal subclavian artery. Normal antegrade flow is therefore up each vertebral artery and into the basilic artery to the brain. When there is disease in the proximal subclavian artery (Figure B.3b) the pressure drop across the stenosis makes the pressure at the origin of the left vertebral artery less than that in the right vertebral or basilic arteries. The path of least resistance to the left arm is then up the right vertebral artery and down the left vertebral artery to the

distal subclavian artery. This phenomenon is known as subclavian steal since the subclavian artery is stealing blood from the vertebral artery. The size of the pressure drop across the stenosis depends on the velocity of blood. This will be greatest during systole and so with a moderate stenosis flow is only reversed during the systolic peak. It is then known as **transient steal**. Figure B.4 shows the sequence of vertebral waveforms obtained as disease in the proximal subclavian artery increases from normal to complete occlusion.

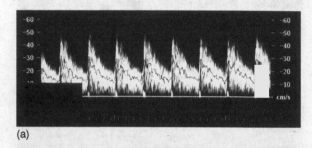

(a)

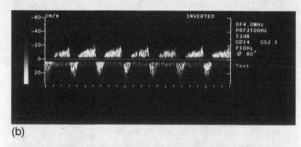

(b)

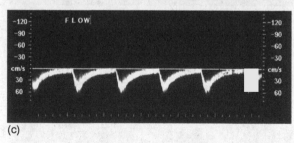

(c)

Figure B.4 – Vertebral artery waveforms: (a) normal waveform; (b) waveform with transient subclavian steal. The velocity becomes negative over the systolic peak when pressure across a subclavian stenosis drops below that in the vertebrobasilar arteries; (c) full steal producing retrograde flow due to proximal subclavian occlusion.

Development of turbulence

Figure B.5 shows the development of turbulence in a damped waveform. There was severe proximal disease causing the waveform to become damped. The flow

Figure B.3 – Pressure changes causing subclavian steal: (a) normal flow pattern; (b) retrograde flow in the left vertebral artery due to proximal subclavian stenosis.

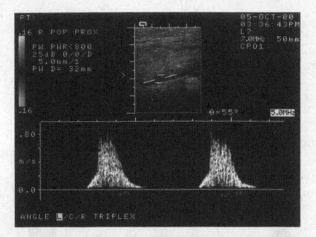

Figure B.5 – Damped waveform showing sharp transition from laminar to turbulent flow.

then encountered further disease in the popliteal artery. As the flow slowly accelerates we see a period of laminar flow giving the waveform a smooth outline. The flow then reaches a velocity where there is a sudden transition to disturbed turbulent flow which continues as the flow slows towards the end of systole.

Carotid flow with aortic valve regurgitation

Figure B.6 shows a common carotid waveform with very low diastolic flow. A low diastolic flow is often seen when the ipsilateral internal carotid artery is occluded producing a high distal resistance. However,

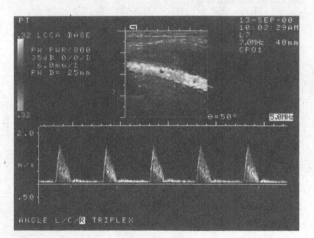

Figure B.6 – Common carotid waveform showing the presence of aortic valve regurgitation reducing reflected wave and diastolic flow.

in this patient the low diastolic flow was seen throughout both left and right carotid arteries. There is also a reduction in the prominence of the notch normally seen on the descending slope of the systolic peak, caused by the reflected wave from the aortic bifurcation. Both changes from normality are caused by aortic valve regurgitation during diastole. This causes a large drop in diastolic pressure and a consequent reduction in diastolic flow seen in both carotid arteries.

Carotid dissection

Figure B.7b shows an unusual waveform seen in the internal carotid artery of a 12-year-old girl who had crawled under a fence and then collapsed when she got up. The waveform results from a carotid dissection in which an intimal flap has become detached from the vessel wall distal to the point of observation. As systolic flow begins, the velocity rises with its usual rapidity but is almost immediately cut off as the intimal flap acts as a valve occluding the vessel. This gives rise to the very abrupt systolic spike with no further flow in diastole. The patient was treated conservatively and by 7 months a normal carotid waveform was seen.

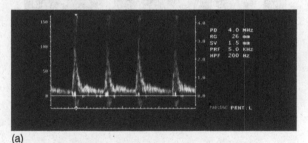

(a)

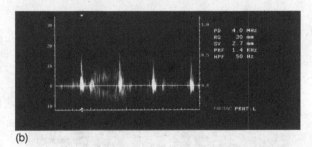

(b)

Figure B.7 – Waveforms obtained from a 12-year-old girl with carotid dissection in the distal internal carotid artery: (a) common carotid artery and (b) internal carotid artery.

APPENDIX C: REFERENCE WAVEFORMS

A set of reference waveforms from a younger normal subject is shown. There may be some variation in waveforms obtained from other normals; in particular the effects of ageing will be seen as indicated in Chapter 6

(Figure 6.31). Any normal waveform should demonstrate the essential shape of the waveforms shown here. An electrocardiogram trace is included so the timing relative to cardiac activity can be seen.

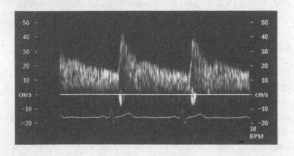

Vertebral artery

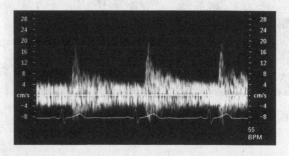

Supertrochlear artery

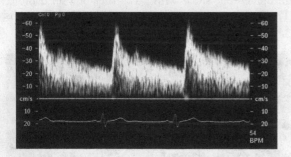

Distal internal carotid artery

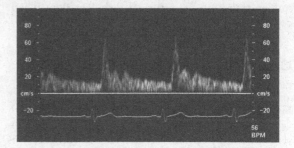

Superficial temporal artery

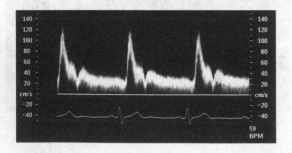

Common carotid artery

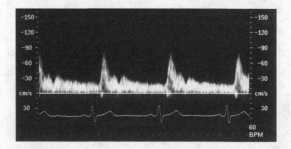

External carotid artery

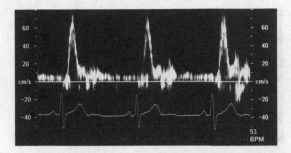

Innominate artery

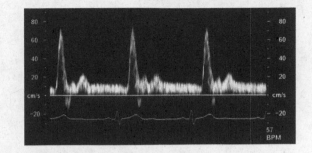

Brachial artery

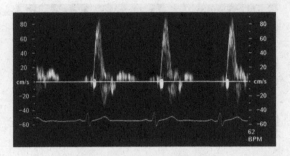

Proximal subclavian artery

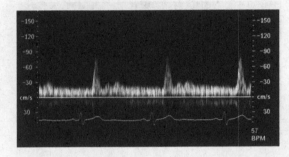

Radial artery at the wrist

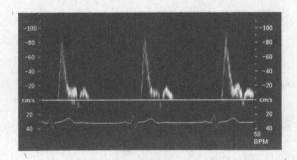

Axillary artery

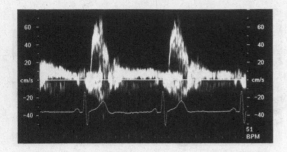

Ascending aorta

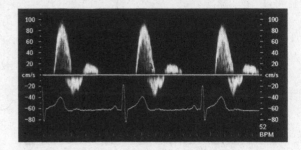

Common femoral artery

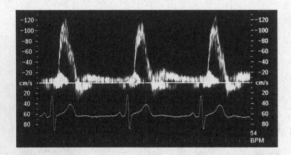

Descending thoracic aorta

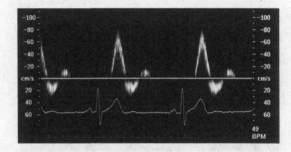

Proximal superficial femoral artery

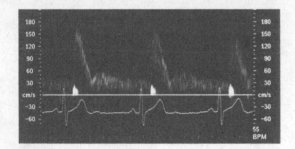

Abdominal aorta

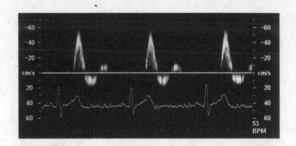

Distal popliteal artery

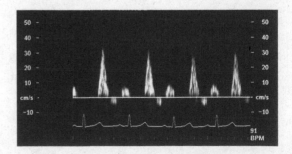

Posterior tibial artery at the ankle

APPENDIX D:
ADDITIONAL DATA

Table D.1 – Typical harmonics for flow and pressure in the ascending aorta of man[1]

Harmonic number	Frequency (Hz)	Flow Modulus (ml s^{-1})	Flow Phase (rad)	Pressure Modulus (mmHg)	Pressure Phase (rad)
0	0	110	–	85	–
1	1.25	202	−0.78	18.6	−1.67
2	2.5	157	−1.50	8.6	−2.25
3	3.75	103	−2.11	5.1	−2.61
4	5	62	−2.46	2.9	−3.12
5	6.25	47	−2.59	1.3	−2.91
6	7.5	42	−2.91	1.4	−2.81
7	8.75	31	2.92	1.2	2.93
8	10	19	2.66	0.4	−2.54
9	11.25	15	2.73	0.6	−2.87
10	12.5	15	2.42	0.6	2.87

Table D.2 – Radial pulsation and pressure–strain modulus E_p in human arteries[2]

Artery	Diameter (cm)	$D_s - D_d$ (cm)	Pressure (mmHg)	Radial pulsation (%)	E_p (× 10^3 Nm^{-2})
Ascending aorta	32.3	2.2	124/80	± 3.4	88
Abdominal aorta	15.5	1.5	117/70	± 4.8	70
Carotid artery	7.1	0.64	117/70	± 4.5	70
Brachial artery	3.6	0.24	116/69	± 3.3	94
Femoral artery	8.1	0.45	116/68	± 0.28	115

References

1. Milnor WR. *Hemodynamics*. Baltimore: Williams & Wilkins, 1982.

2. Nichols WW, O'Rourke MF. *Mcdonald's Blood Flow in Arteries*, 4th edn. London: Arnold, 1998.

INDEX FOR CARDIOVASCULAR HAEMODYNAMICS AND DOPPLER WAVEFORMS EXPLAINED

Printed in the United States
By Bookmasters